Heal Yourself

Practical methods on how to heal yourself
from any disease using the power of the
subconscious mind and natural medicine

Heal Yourself

Practical methods on how to heal yourself
from any disease using the power of the
subconscious mind and natural medicine

Max Corradi

(MBRCP, MISOHH, Hons)

AYNI
BOOKS

Winchester, UK
Washington, USA

First published by Ayni Books, 2013
Ayni Books is an imprint of John Hunt Publishing Ltd., Laurel House, Station Approach,
Alresford, Hants, SO24 9JH, UK
office1@jhpbooks.net
www.johnhuntpublishing.com
www.ayni-books.com

For distributor details and how to order please visit the 'Ordering' section on our website.

A CIP catalogue record for this book is available from the British Library.

Design: Lee Nash

Front cover image artwork "Sky Lotus Tree" by the artist Cristina Jimenez Rodriguez

Contact: kristinajr.cristina@gmail.com

Printed and bound by CPI Group (UK) Ltd, Croydon, CR0 4YY

We operate a distinctive and ethical publishing philosophy in all
areas of our business, from our global network of authors to
production and worldwide distribution.

CONTENTS

This book is dedicated to all my kind teachers, and to all those who are suffering from illnesses and poverty. This book has been inspired by the teachings of the Buddha and Christ, and the writings of William Walker Atkinson, Thomas Troward, Giordano Bruno, Baron Eugene Fersen, Thomas Hamblin, Florence Shinn, Genevieve Behrend, Neville Goddard, Paracelsus, Samuel Hahnemann, James Tyler Kent, Hans-Heinrich Reckeweg, Professor Ivo Bianchi, Dr. Jerome Malzac and Dr. Jo Sorrentino.

Introduction

Health is contagious as well as Disease.
William Walker Atkinson

The subject of this book is healing and self-help.

The book includes two different healing approaches using the subconscious mind and natural medicine. The first part gives you a complete list and explanation of useful healing methods using the most powerful of all human beings resources which is the subconscious mind. You will learn how powerful the mind is in every process of healing, and you will learn how to work with those natural and fundamental laws of mind and nature like the Law of Cause and Effect and the Law of Vibration. Through these simple but effective methods you will be able to reprogram your subconscious mind.

In Part 2 the book covers a great deal of useful information about natural medicine like phytotherapy, homeopathy, advanced complex homeopathy, homotoxicology, micotherapy, nutrition and low dose embryo therapy for cancer. It includes a comprehensive list of natural medicine protocols for a wide variety of health conditions and a compendium of low dose homeopathic hormones, cytokines and growth factors with their main indications.

Important Disclaimer:
The knowledge presented in this book is intended to complement medical treatment not to replace conventional medicine or the advice of your doctor. Always seek professional help.
NOTHING CONTAINED IN THIS BOOK IS INTENDED TO BE NOR CAN IT BE TAKEN FOR MEDICAL DIAGNOSIS OR TREATMENT.

Part 1

The mind is the king of healers

Mind is the chief and it is swift. Mind is the forerunner of all things.
Udanavarga Sutra – The Buddha

Chapter I

The conscious and the subconscious mind

The first aspect of our consciousness or mind is the conscious mind or objective mind. It is the mind which knows the objects of the senses and perceives its own thoughts and emotions. It is also that aspect of the mind that is able to reason and discriminate.

If we use it with the presence of awareness it becomes the guardian at the door of the subconscious mind, ensuring that only wanted and empowering messages are allowed through as it is only through the conscious mind that we can access the subconscious.

The subconscious mind or unconscious mind on the other hand is an incredibly powerful program that runs every aspect of our life automatically and without any need for our conscious input.

In the subconscious mind are stored all our beliefs about reality and all the habitual tendencies which manifest as intuitions, tendencies to feel in a certain way, to behave in a certain way, to react in a certain way, basically all aspects of our waking and dream life.

Let's take a closer look at some of the attributes of the subconscious mind and understand how it works.

First the subconscious mind cannot distinguish between what is real and what is imagined; it follows orders by acting on whatever is fed to it. It responds with instincts and habits which are manifested into our waking lives and dreams.

The subconscious mind does not process negatives. For this reason, all affirmations, statements and visualizations must affirm the positive.

The subconscious represses memories with unresolved negative emotions. The memories get buried, yet the beliefs, feelings and emotions associated with them will still control our reactions.

The subconscious works with symbols and associations, and it records everything in first person. For example whenever we criticize, judge and project negative thoughts and feelings onto others, we experience the negativity as our own.

It also works on the principle of least effort by following the path of least resistance. **Without a proper and purposeful direction from our conscious mind, it follows the easiest, but sometimes more negative path of our habitual tendencies.**

There is no future or past in the subconscious mind; since it can only process the present time, all stored experiences are processed in the ever present NOW of our life. As we have seen the whole of mind can be compared to an iceberg floating in the ocean. Consciousness is the tip of the iceberg, consisting of information and stimuli of which we are aware. The subconscious is the deep underside of the mind, recording and processing information.

On the more physical side, a developing brain can be compared to an onion. Each layer, larger than the other, growing and forming new neuro pathways able to direct the body's reflexive and voluntary movement, memory, thought and emotional behavior until there is a vast data bank of unconscious skills, abilities and emotions and habitual tendencies.

Simply put, any thought, message, emotion or order that is given to the subconscious often enough and convincingly enough will, in time, be accepted as truth and consistently be carried out with exact precision irrespective of whether it is for our benefit or not. Another important thing is that the subconscious mind is neutral in nature, and this means that it cannot reason or distinguish between positive and negative. In other words, anything we think or intend and do will leave a trace, or become a cause so to speak for its subsequent manifestation as anything in our life, whether it is for our benefit or harm.

Among the several ways to consciously reprogram the subconscious mind, the quickest and most effective ones are the statements or self-suggestions and the creative visualizations which we will discuss later.

When reprogramming your subconscious mind and changing your underlying habits, you will know to what degree your underlying negative beliefs have been replaced by the new beliefs by checking how much willpower you have to use to do something that serves your positive intention. If you have to use a great deal of willpower then there is probably still a major conflict between your positive intention and the underlying negative habit. Anything you do, say or think that is aligned with your beliefs, whether positive or negative, requires not much willpower and is effortless. Willpower is the domain of the conscious mind whereas our aim is to transform our positive thought-intentions and actions into habits of the subconscious mind.

Chapter 2

Cause and effect and positive thinking

Suggestions for Practical Application

When you treat a disease, first treat the mind.
Chen Jen

Our physical health and obviously our mental health are for the most part dominated by our mind as in our dominant thoughts and emotions. If we maintain a mental peaceful attitude of joyful health, strength and fearlessness, this will manifest accordingly on the physical plane.

But if we go about with a mind filled with ideas and thoughts of a depressing and angry nature our body-mind will likewise respond sooner or later.

Thoughts and emotions always precede actions of voice and body; therefore we should place more emphasis on our thoughts and emotions if we want to have visible effects in our lives.

Every action and feeling is preceded by a thought, and right thinking begins with the words we say to ourselves.

As you sow, you shall reap.
Galatians 6:7

In the Bible the so-called Eastern Law of Karma or Cause and Effect is mentioned in just a few words with exactly the same meaning. We also find it in the Jewish Kabbalah as *Tikune*, the ancient Egyptians called it *Maat* and the ancient Greeks called it *Heimarmene*.

Although there are many laws in the universe, this is the most important Law because it rules all planes of reality.

Karma is mainly the urge or the will to act in a certain way and this is usually started at the level of an intention with a specific motivation or intended result. Thoughts and intentions are like seeds and they produce effects not only on the mind level, by producing more like-minded thoughts, but also on an emotional and physical level. When we talk about physical and verbal actions, these are usually started with mental urges, they have a mental cause.

Every one of our thoughts, words or actions set a specific chain of causation in motion which will come to materialize over time into certain effects, and this is always started at the level of mind with our intentions and aims, as we are told by the Hermetic axiom of the Principle of Correspondence:

As above so below, as below so above.

Although the Law of Cause and Effect applies to all levels of existence, and, as we shall see later, time and space are relative concepts, since our lives are tightly bound by our concept of time and space there is usually a time gap between the cause and the eventual effect which always depends on other secondary conditions to manifest.

To illustrate the Law of Cause and Effect in relation to time the Buddha said:

Truly, an evil deed committed does not immediately bear fruit, like milk that does not turn sour all at once. But smoldering, it follows the fool like fire covered by ashes.

As the Law of Cause and Effect is very difficult to comprehend in full (it will be the subject of my next book on the Seven Hermetic Principles), we shall limit by saying that one cause can produce many effects, many causes can produce one effect, that the effect is never lost with the passing of time unless it is counteracted by an opposite cause and that effects become causes reinforcing the original causes, which will then produce more effects and so on in a chain of causation extending *ad infinitum.*

Health and ease is our birthright, and since effects can produce new causes, and everything starts at the level of mind, the *"as above"* level of the axiom so to speak, we can work with the Law of Cause and Effect, by stating and visualizing our goal or outcome of full health and recovery already a reality in the ever present NOW, as this statement will set in motion a new chain of causation which will eventually result in health and vigor on all planes of existence, i.e. mind, energy and physical.

It is particularly important that we should not think of ourselves in recovery in a distant future when we use these methods, **otherwise our focus of perception would be on the present lack of health**, therefore reinforcing our disease state and postponing our recovery.

If a thing is true at all, there is a way in which it is true throughout the universe. Remember that the power of thought and intentions works by absolutely scientific principles. These principles are expressed in the language of the statement:

As a man thinketh in his heart, so is he.

Note: Law of attraction and Law of Cause and Effect clarification

Many people might say that what I'm presenting here is similar to what nowadays is sold as the law of attraction due to the success of the movie *The Secret*.

Let me clarify this before we move forward. The term "law of attraction" was coined by the great writer and occultist William Walker Atkinson in 1906 in his published book *Thought Vibration or the Law of Attraction in the Thought World*.

But in this and other books, Atkinson clearly states the following about the law of attraction and materialization:

9

They are a part of the working of the law of Cause and Effect in its phase of thought attraction.

So there is no separate law of attraction, as in reality the law of attraction is but one phase, or we could also say, the visible manifestation of the working and interaction of the Law of Cause and Effect and the Law of Vibration, another Hermetic Law. Further proof of this is that there is no separate law of attraction in the seven Hermetic Laws or Principles of ancient Hermetic Philosophy from which Atkinson and all the other New Thought writers of the last century drew their ideas and realizations.

The seven Hermetic Laws or Principles of the Universe are: The Principle of Mind (All is Mind), the Principle of Correspondence, the Principle of Vibration, the Principle of Polarity, the Principle of Rhythm, the Principle of Cause and Effect, the Principle of Gender.

The axiom of the proponents of the law of attraction *'like attracts like'* still remains valid on all planes of mind, energy and physical reality through the working and interaction of the Law of Cause and Effect and the Law of Vibration creating the conditions for various events to manifest first in the mind and then in the energetic and physical planes in a *'like attracts like'* fashion.

We must bear in mind that these unchangeable Laws are not exclusive of each other but are all working in synergy throughout the universe in the same way as the law of gravity is not exclusive of the law of lift on the physical plane.

Although in this book we cannot explain in depth the working of these seven Laws (see my next book on the Seven Hermetic Laws), suffice to say we can use the laws of nature, but we cannot alter them. By opposing any natural law we place ourselves in an inverted position with regard to it and, therefore, it appears as though the law itself is working against us with a definite purpose. But this inversion is entirely caused by ourselves, and not from any change in the action of the law.

Mind precedes all mental states. Mind is their chief; they are all mind-wrought. If with an impure mind a person speaks or acts, suffering follows him like the wheel that follows the foot of the ox. Dhammapada – The Buddha

Chapter 3

Self healing statements

The mind is the key to the man.
James Tyler Kent

Reestablishing a link to health and recovery starts by saying in your mind the following statements, repeating them and feeling their actuality. This must be done in a relaxed and silent environment first, best in the morning and evening before and after the daily activities, but there is no limitation, you can do it as much as you want; the important thing is to FEEL and believe what you are mentally saying. Later we will combine them with the creative visualizations to have a more powerful effect. You might want to concentrate more on the easy ones at first, the ones which resonate more with you, and later move on to the more difficult ones, the ones for which you feel more resistance.

I can be what I will myself to be.

This affirmation gives us a sense of power over our present circumstances and is a good one to start with, as usually during an illness we often feel powerless and discouraged.

I am fearless – absolutely fearless and relaxed.

This statement relieves us from the strong fears we have to deal with, like the fear of pain and of not recovering.

I am getting strong and well – I am manifesting health. I radiate hope, cheerfulness and joy.

This statement goes to the heart of the matter as it can be used also to alter our mood if we are often feeling depressed or sad, and is also very powerful in physical illnesses as it is more difficult to heal ourselves when we feel hopeless and depressed.

Loving light floods my mind and body with health and strength, and every cell is filled with healing light.

This statement is important as it changes our fixation on the illness by putting a cause and therefore giving reality to its opposite, which is health and positive energy.

I'm grateful for all the good things that have already manifested in my life and the ones which are about to manifest, especially the health and the energy of health.

Appreciation and gratefulness as well as love are the most powerful emotions for living a healthy and joyful life. We should be grateful first for all the good things which we have experienced in our life, but also for all the ones that are going to manifest because we are planting the seeds for them to manifest; this is also the base for developing faith.

I forgive everyone and everyone forgives me.

Usually we have a very deep ingrained guilt towards ourselves and hatred towards others for whatever reasons. If we want to be well, healthy and joyful we must let go of all hatred and guilt; there is no room for them in a healthy life.

How to change negative feeling moods into positive.
As we have seen, one of the seven Hermetic Laws or Principles of the universe is the Law of Vibration which states that everything manifests as a rate of vibration.

Another Principle is the Law of Polarity which states that everything has two poles, everything has its pair of opposites and that opposites are identical in nature but different in degree, depending on the rate of vibration. The higher the vibration, the higher the position in the scale. The positive pole always dominates the negative because of the tendency of nature to go in the direction of the dominant activity of the positive pole.

If you find yourself in an undesirable mood or you want to overcome a negative quality, concentrate upon the positive pole of that same quality or mood, and the vibrations will gradually change from negative to positive, until finally you will become polarized on the positive pole instead of the negative.

Through the use of the statements and visualizations, which will be explained later, you will be able to change your mental vibrations and master your moods.

Note: Always make positive suggestions or affirmations. For instance, do not say: "I'm not ill." But on the contrary say, "I'm Strong" or "I'm healthy." The reason lies in the fact that by repeating the word of the thing you would deny, you really affirm its existence, and direct the mind to it as the mind is always inclusive.

Remember that it is your freedom to choose just what you want to think.

Chapter 4

Visualization and creative Imagination

Imagination is more important than knowledge for knowledge is limited to all we now know and understand, while imagination embraces the entire world and all there ever will be to know and understand. 'Logic' will get you from A to B. Imagination will take you everywhere...
Albert Einstein

Creative visualization is the creative process employed by forming and holding a mental image of the conditions as you wish them to be in actuality. The mental image tends to create an objective form and existence; it is the mental pattern around which the material conditions tend to group themselves. It is the seed-form of the thing itself.

Mastering creative visualization grants you direct control over your thoughts at the subconscious level. While there are several ways to reprogram the subconscious mind, visualization is the most effective and its results the most rapid.

The creative power of any mental image is determined by how often you imagine it and by the strength of the feelings or emotions associated with it.

By planting seeds of recovery in the subconscious mind, we are planting the possibility of recovery which in due time will become an actuality for our conscious mind through a reprogramming process of our subconscious.

How is this possible? As we have already seen, health and ease is our birthright; and since everything starts at the level of mind, we can work with the laws of nature by stating and visualizing our goal or outcome of full health and recovery as already a reality in the ever present NOW, as this will set in motion a new chain of causation which will eventually result in our feeling and manifestation of health.

We shall not worry about how our recovery is going to manifest, that's not our job, the recovery will manifest in its own manner and following its own routes; we will maybe be offered the right and most effective therapy among many, or we will meet the right doctor which best understands what we need, we will have an intuition regarding the right therapy to follow, and so on. Most importantly, our mind will be in a better mood, we will have the strength to carry on with whatever therapies we are doing and we will take the right decisions for ourselves without doubt or hesitation. We will not be passive and hopeless, but cheerful and active in whatever situation.

We shouldn't feel attachment to the outcome, as attachment is based on doubt; on the other hand detachment is based on faith, confidence and certainty of the outcome.

Note: Although the statements and the visualizations I'm presenting are mainly for the restoration of health, as this is the subject of this book, you can adapt them and use them for any positive aim in your life, like creating more abundance for yourself and others or improving your relationships etc.

Creative visualization is not daydreaming

Some people might object that creative visualizations are like daydreaming and therefore a waste of time.

To this I reply that daydreaming is a waste of time and energy, in fact in daydreaming we dissipate our mind-energy with no effect at all. In creative visualization, on the contrary, we focus our mind-energy like a magnifying glass for a specific aim, our recovery and full restoration of health and therefore achieve our goal. Moreover, in creative visualization we focus on the outcome as already an actuality in the ever present now and not as something happening in a distant future.

Another difference between creative visualization and

daydreaming is that in creative visualization there is no doubt, as in daydreaming where we project a desire into a future which will never come. Instead in creative visualization we know without doubt that what we intend will manifest because we are putting the causes for its manifestation.

The visualizations

You can do the visualizations anytime but at least in the morning and in the evening before going to sleep for about 15 minutes, but you must try to be present and watch your mind during the rest of the day; don't let the doubt and the habitual negative patterns jeopardize your positive work. You can't expect to be positive for 30 minutes a day and angry and depressed the rest of the day and at the same time expect positive results; that would be like planting seeds of one kind and expecting fruits of another; remember all is cause and effect.

If you are using these visualizations and you are facing a long-term illness or you feel a lot of pain, remember not to force your mind, be gentle on yourself, acknowledge how you feel but at the same time take the attention away from the pain to your visualizations and statements, knowing that you are planting the seeds in your mind which will then have an effect sooner or later. The important thing is not to dwell and put attention on the lack of health; just acknowledge it and focus on your visualizations at least for the time you have set for it.

Here we combine the visualizations and repeat the statements to ourselves mentally to reinforce our visualized objective.

Visualization one: Imagine yourself performing an activity which you would normally feel fear for, but in this case see yourself as completely relaxed and acting fearlessly, having moral and physical courage, and driving away any worry. We are using a symbol to acquire and develop certain qualities associated with that symbol.

Repeat to yourself: I am fearless – absolutely fearless and relaxed.

Visualization two: Visualize yourself as healthy, joyful and in full strength, doing any activities that please you like sports, or any social activities, something which brings good feelings by thinking of it. It would have to be something which you think of as possible and pleasant but not strenuous.

Repeat to yourself: I am getting strong and well – I am manifesting health. I radiate hope, cheerfulness and joy.

Visualization three: Imagine soothing white or blue light surrounding you and flowing into your body; your body now is flooded with light, in fact it is now a vibrant and healthy light body; all your cells are nourished with healing and soothing light.

Repeat to yourself: Loving light floods my mind and body with health and strength, every cell is filled with healing light, health is restored.

Visualization four: Imagine loving and forgiving white light expanding from you and going to all the people you have a connection with, relatives, friends and enemies, then imagine this white loving and forgiving light coming back to you and making you feel at peace and joyful.

Repeat to yourself: I forgive everyone and everyone forgives me.

In conclusion see yourself in your 'mind's eye' as you wish yourself to be: healthy, in full strength with a joyful poise. From time to time you can talk to yourself and tell your mind what you expect it to do for you, taking hold of the physical body and building up new cells and tissue and discarding the old worn-out and diseased cells. We will cover this type of healing method more in depth in Chapter 8.

Chapter 5

Prayer and the power of mind

If you are not a spiritual or religious person you can skip this section; but if you are a spiritual person you might want to use prayer, and in this case there is also a method to follow.

You can combine the prayers with the visualizations, thinking that the blessing lights are coming from your holy object of refuge, of whatever faith it might be.

In prayer for a change in conditions, physical or mental for yourself or another, bear in mind that the fundamental necessity for the answer to prayer is the understanding of the Bible statement:

Whatsoever things you ask for when you pray, *believe that you receive them,* **and you shall have them.**
Mark 11:24

These are the words of Christ and are mainly related with what we call faith.

What is faith?

Faith is the substance of things hoped for, the evidence of things not seen.
Hebrews 11:1

In the words of Francis Shinn:

Hope looks forward; Faith knows it has already received.

In our modern society we call this confidence, we feel absolutely confident in the answer to our prayer.

This is not as difficult as it appears on the surface, once you realize that everything has its origin in the mind, and that which you seek outwardly, you already possess. Your thoughts, visualizations and prayers of recovery and health constitute the origin or cause in the ever present now of the subconscious mind, and causes produce effects.

You can close your meditation, visualizations and prayer with the happy assurance that your mind is a center of divine operation.

Chapter 6

Dieting and addictions

The only reason most diets fail is because of the negative underlying belief stored in the subconscious. If you are following a diet with a belief such as "I am fat" or "I will always be fat" or "I tried everything and nothing works", then no diet or exercise regime will be accomplished with permanent success if that belief remains unchanged. Sooner or later, you will take actions to fulfill that negative belief again. The decision to go on a diet as a fulfillment of the negative "I am fat" belief will sabotage your efforts.

Once you change the negative belief associated with that negative habit, then changing the actual habits will come far more easily and the outcome will also follow.

In this case you can use the statement **"I am healthy and slim"** and adopt the following creative visualizations:

You could either start by focusing and visualizing yourself as slim, or pick a physical activity that you would like to complete if you were slim or that would cause you to become slim instead. At some point you will find yourself adopting new healthy eating and exercise habits without any conscious effort.

You will soon find that your thoughts and actions in your waking life will begin to reflect your new beliefs until such time that they too become habitual in nature.

Addictions

Addictions can take almost any form and shape, but no matter how they manifest, all addictions have one thing in common: they are based on an underlying craving for fulfillment and the negative beliefs and habitual tendencies stored in the subconscious mind related to the object of craving.

The first thing to do is to look at the messages that have been implanted into the subconscious mind, because these are the messages that we have to erase. For example if you are a smoker, a negative habitual tendency based on that craving is stored in the subconscious mind that actually tells the body that it needs to have nicotine and this is the sort of dangerous association that we have to be aware of and try to change.

Start by repeating the following statements:

I deny the power of... such and such addiction... over my free will.
I'm free, completely free from... such and such addiction.
I'm free to choose my desires to my best interest.

In addition to the statements you could visualize and see yourself in a typical situation but free of the object of addiction.

For example if you are a smoker and wish to quit, you could see yourself at a bar with friends perfectly fulfilled without the need to smoke. Or you could visualize refusing a cigarette offer without any effort.

The important thing is to associate to such addiction-free visualization and statements a feeling of complete fulfillment and freedom.

As we have seen the subconscious is a servant of the conscious mind. It follows orders by acting on whatever is fed to it. It cannot distinguish between what is real and what is imagined. Moreover the subconscious mind works with symbols, associations and metaphors, therefore it can be easily reprogrammed.

On the more physical level you can follow the Biotherapies laid out in Part 2 of this book, starting with a deep detoxification and drainage treatment and a full support of the PNEI system.

Chapter 7

Prana healing or healing through breathing

Different self healing methods using the mind and breathing

There are also different methods of healing using visualization along with the breathing. This form of healing uses what in general is called Prana.

Prana is a Sanskrit word which means 'Vital Force' or 'Vital Energy'.

The Chinese call it Chi or Qi and the Japanese Ki. Prana is very much connected to our breathing as breathing is also life, therefore in Prana healing we use visualizations along with the breathing in order to achieve the desired outcome.

I will only outline three basic forms of Pranic self healing:

General self healing, inhibiting pain and recharging yourself.

Note: Never force your breathing, but let it flow in and out effortlessly.

General self healing

Lying in a relaxed condition, as you breathe in imagine the Prana flowing into you; with the exhalation send the Prana to the affected part for the purpose of stimulating or healing it. Vary this occasionally by exhaling, with the intent that the diseased condition be forced out and disappear. You can also use the hands in this method by passing them down the body from the head to the affected part. In using the hands in healing yourself always hold the mental image that the Prana is flowing down the arm and through the fingertips into the body, thus reaching the affected part and healing it.

During the exhalation feel that the Prana or vital energy is being distributed all over the body, to every organ and part, to

23

every muscle, to cells, nerves, arteries and veins; from the top of your head to the soles of your feet, invigorating, strengthening and stimulating every part.

You can also try to form a mental picture of the inflowing Prana, coming in through the lungs and being taken up by the solar plexus, then with the exhaling effort, being sent to all parts of the system, down to the fingertips and down to the toes.

The most essential self healing method is to practice deep breathing and think and feel that you are drawing in health and strength and breathing out the old diseased conditions.

Healing Painful conditions

Lying down or sitting, as before, breathe in and imagine the Prana flowing into you, thinking that you are inhaling Prana. Then when you exhale, send the Prana to the painful part to reestablish the circulation and healing it. Then inhale more Prana for the purpose of driving out the painful condition; then exhale, holding the thought that you are driving out the pain. Alternate the two mental visualizations, and with one exhalation stimulate or heal the part and with the next drive out the pain. You can do this seven times, then rest. Then start again until relief comes. If the hand is placed over the painful part, you may get quicker results by sending the current of Prana down the arm and into the painful part.

Recharging Yourself

If you feel that your vital energy is low or you feel always tired, there is a method which is quite useful in recharging yourself using a specific position called 'the Star' position.

It's a very simple exercise which enables you to make contact with the universal life force or energy.

The Star Exercise

Take a position of a 5-pointed star, by standing straight, legs apart but not too far from each other, arms stretched on either side on a level with the shoulders, head straight looking in front and the palm of the left hand should be turned up slightly curved facing the sky as in receiving and the right hand turned down facing the earth.

The image resembles a 5-pointed star and also somewhat the famous drawing by Leonardo da Vinci, *Vitruvian Man,* where there are two identical men inside a circle.

There is no need to visualize anything in this case but just to feel the force of energy flowing through you, coming from above in the left palm, circulating the body, penetrating every cell, storing in the solar plexus and flowing out to the earth from the right palm.

We take the blessing from above, and we give blessing to what is below; in this way the circle is complete.

There are two different sensations, one of heaviness on the left hand due to the energy flowing in, and tingling on the fingers of the right hand.

You should do this exercise for about 3 to 5 minutes in the morning after getting up and in the evening before going to sleep, preferably in the open air; never force the position but slowly build your capacity to hold the position in a relaxed manner. You should never do it after any meal as you might develop nausea due to a strong magnetic current flowing through the digestive tract.

Chapter 8

Suggestive Healing

The central theory around suggestive healing is that the disease is a mental condition, but not only a condition in the central mind, but also in the mind of the different cells and the organs. The theory of the cure is that thought suggestion overcomes the rebellious mind in the cells and organs, and forces it to resume its normal action.

This form of healing is based on the supposition that all cells have a kind of basic intelligence as part of the whole mind, and therefore can be told and trained. You are not using mind against matter, but mind to train mind, the central conscious mind to train the particular cell mind. There is no dead matter in a living body, mind is in every part and cells; do not forget this, because it underlies the whole system of this type of treatment.

Tell the mind of the cells or organs what it must do, talk to it just as you would to a child that was not doing what it should; reason with it, and lead or drive it along.

Remember that the cell's mind does not understand the words you say as it doesn't have such knowledge, but it understands the thoughts and feelings that lie behind the words, and will respond to them. The words only serve to help you to form your thoughts clearly. Words are symbols of thoughts.

Point out to the mind of the organs or cells just what you expect it to do, and you will be surprised at how readily it will follow your directions.

Examples of Suggestive Healing

Start by directing your thoughts to the mind in the part or organ that needs to be healed, by addressing it positively, either by uttering the actual words or by speaking them mentally. It could be something like this:

Dear… (organ or part), you are not behaving well, you know better, and I expect you to do better, you must and will do better. You must bring about normal and healthy conditions. I expect you to do the right work to restore health.

This is just an example, and you can customize the words as you please, the important thing is that you approach your mind in a kind but firm way, not begging but more like a kind of soft order.

I'm going to give just a few examples of different conditions that can be treated with this approach. The treatment should last about five to ten minutes depending on the condition.

Heart

Start by lying down on your back if you can or sitting down.

The heart is the most intelligent of the organs, and it has a higher grade of mind in it than any other organs apart from the brain. This heart mind will respond readily to loving, gentle and kind instructions. In the case the heart is palpitating or beating irregularly, place the hand gently over the chest, and say kindly, "Heart mind, quiet down, quiet, quiet, act regularly, and quietly, steady, steady," etc. You will find that the palpitation will gradually quiet down and the heart's action will become steady and regular.

Stomach

Start by giving the stomach several quick but gentle taps or pats of the hand or placing the hand over it and say:

Dear stomach mind, I want you to begin to function properly, and make my stomach strong, healthy, and active. You must digest the food properly, and nourish the whole body. You must relieve the indigestion.

You need not repeat these exact words, as you may add or vary them. The main thing is to tell the stomach mind what you expect it to do, and what you want it to bring about. You will be surprised at the intelligence displayed by the mind addressed, and how quickly it begins to act upon your instructions.

Liver

Treat the liver in a similar manner to the stomach. The liver, however, being a more dull or stubborn organ, must be spoken to sharply and positively. The liver cannot be persuaded, it must be driven like a mule. Give the liver instructions to function properly, to detoxify properly your blood, to secrete the proper amount of bile, to let the bile flow freely and perform its work, and if you overindulge in toxic substances you can also excuse yourself for having done so.

Kidneys

The kidneys are treated in a similar manner to the liver. Tap them smartly with the fingers, several times, and then tell them to do their work properly, and naturally. In cases where you urinate too frequently, instruct the kidneys and bladder to, *"Slow down,"* and endeavor to reduce the urination gradually.

Circulation

Say to the mind of the arteries and veins: *"Flow freely, and equally, steadily and constantly; flow, circulate, flow."*

Female related conditions

In case of profuse flow, add the words: *"Slow down, slow down the flow,"* etc. In the case of scant flow, *"Flow, circulate, flow."*

Headaches

Headaches are treated by first treating the stomach and liver, and then by equalizing the circulation, and then giving local treatments to the head, placing the hand to the affected part of the head saying: *"Quiet down, now, easy, easy, rest, rest..."* etc.

These are just a few examples; in a nutshell you must tell the mind of the parts, cells or organs what they must do to heal the health condition, remembering always that you are talking to the mind of the organs and not to dead matter.

Chapter 9

Concluding advice

I want to close Part 1 with a last advice which comes from the Tibetan culture. In Tibet it is a custom, in order to prolong and have a healthier life, to save other forms of life which are destined to be killed, or are suffering imminent death. Usually this would be animals which are destined to be slaughtered but can also be small insects or any animal we might find in cities or rural areas which might be suffering in some way.

I consider this a sound attitude based on love and compassion, based on the Law of Cause and Effect and the interdependence of all life on earth.

If you don't have chances to save animals but you like the idea of doing so, you can sponsor with an offering the "Animal Liberation Fund" at this website address: http://www.fpmt. org/projects/fpmt/alf.html

Where there is a mind, there are feelings such as pain, pleasure, and joy. No sentient being wants pain; instead all want happiness. Since we all share these feelings at some basic level, we as rational human beings have an obligation to contribute in whatever way we can to the happiness of other species and try our best to relieve their fears and sufferings.
His Holiness the 14th Dalai Lama

Part 2

How to heal yourself using natural medicine

Introduction

In this second part of the book I will present different possible treatments for a wide variety of conditions using herbal remedies and homeopathic remedies combined and integrated in a new form of treatment called Biotherapy. The Biotherapy treatments that I'm going to present can be combined with the self healing methods presented in Part 1 to achieve a quicker recovery.

Note: I want to clarify that I'm not against conventional medicine, when it is needed in life-saving situations and in life-threatening illnesses. In fact in many cases we can combine the conventional Western drugs especially with the homeopathic complex remedies, in order to lower the dose and the frequency of the drugs until they can, in many cases, be stopped altogether.

Unfortunately we see a lot indiscriminate prescription of drugs with so many side effects, even for minor conditions that could be cured easily with natural remedies, and this is a sign of the degenerate times we live in, where profit has become more important than even health.

As in the axiom written on the Temple of Apollo in ancient Greece which said: *"nothing in excess"*, I believe we should never fall into extremes, but use our reasoning mind and sound judgment before we decide the best therapy treatment.

The good physician treats the disease; the great physician treats the patient.
Sir William Osler

Chapter 10

The importance of detoxification and drainage

Any agent, whether physical, chemical or microbial, that adversely modifies or damages a balanced biological system is considered a 'toxin'. Toxins may enter the body from the external environment (exogenous toxins – microbes, viruses, fungi, environmental, chemicals etc) through the gastrointestinal system by ingestion, the respiratory system by inhalation, and the skin by passive absorption or by injection. Toxins may also originate within the body itself (endogenous toxins) as by-products of physiological metabolism (bilirubin, creatinine, lactic acid, etc.) or as metabolites under abnormal metabolic conditions (excess production/degradations of neurotransmitters and hormones, excess free radical formation etc.).

Chemical compounds are currently spread all over the world, even if the chemical was not used in the specific area, due to distribution via the ground water, surface rain and winds. Bioaccumulation of these compounds cause disease in all living beings by disrupting the immune system, the endocrine system and neurological system.

The effects of toxins are documented in a number of diseases, ranging from asthma, allergies, autoimmunity, cancers, cognitive deficit, and obesity.

We can easily say that the ability to detoxify and eliminate toxins is equivalent to the maintenance of health in an organism.

The main organs of detoxification are: the liver and gallbladder, the kidneys, the extracellular matrix (an 'organ' that comprises the layers of tissue between the cells and the regulatory organs), the lymphatic system, the bowels, and the skin.

It should be clear from the above that toxins stored in the body and not eliminated will be detrimental for various reasons and can have a wide range of effects such as fatigue, cognitive deficit, obesity, asthma, allergies, autoimmunity, cancers etc.

Even more important to remember is that without a proper detoxified matrix, due to the toxic overload, any treatment you undertake will be much less effective if at all.

That's why it is so important to detoxify and drain the organism, and this is done by stopping the external supply of toxins, supporting the organs of detoxification and drainage, and stimulating the elimination of toxins from the matrix.

It is often said that a good detoxification and drainage is already half of any treatments.

Note: As we will see later, the only time when is not advisable to do a full detoxification and especially drainage is during cancer treatments where we should instead support the organs of detoxification and work mainly on the PNEI system.

Chapter 11

The PNEI: Psycho-Neuro-Endocrine-Immune System

Psycho-neuro-endocrine-immunology is the study of how psychological factors influence the nervous, hormonal and immune systems and gives clues to how stress affects both our mental and physical being. The comprehension of the constant contact, communication and interdependence of these four systems is the reading key for the identification of physiopathological mechanisms which lie at the heart of many conditions and illnesses.

The ancient concept of *'mens sana in corpore sano'* (a healthy mind in a healthy body) is still very relevant and has been proved by recent discoveries in the field of PNEI. Factors like psychological-behavioral patterns, and, above all, sustained stress can change and alter the immunological answer. However, chronic stress is also involved in pathologies like heart conditions, hypertension, viral and bacteria infections, auto-immune diseases, depression, infertility; basically all the pathologies that afflict our modern society.

Henri Laborit, one of the pioneers of the PNEI theory, has correlated the mind-body relations and has defined the maintenance of the health state not only as internal physiological balance but also in relation to the outside environment. According to Laborit the variation of stressful external circumstances if prolonged can cause an energy imbalance and can determine a lowering of the immune defenses. Psychological factors are the most common trigger of PNEI imbalance. Cortisol and adrenalin are regularly increased in acute states of stress, conditions which when prolonged enough may eventually precipitate resistance of insulin receptors and induce diabetes mellitus. Adrenal exhaustion, hypofunction and consequent hypoglycemia tend to follow the phase of an increased steroid production. Stressful states may also disturb the hypothalamic-pituitary axis, resulting in thyroid problems. In the PNEI vision, the neuroendocrine and immune systems act, respectively, as sense organs in the management of cognitive and non-cognitive stressors. Exposure to repeated cognitive, non-cognitive, physical or environmental psycho-emotional stress of sufficient intensity can cause or exacerbate an imbalance in the formation and metabolism of cerebral chemicals called amines (amines are neurotransmitters like dopamine, serotonin, histamine, noradrenaline involved in mood regulation, attention, appetite control, reward, addiction, inflammation etc). In the treatments chapter I present different low dose biotherapy protocols which work by stimulating or inhibiting psycho-neuro-endocrine-immune processes in order to de-stress and regulate the organism.

Chapter 12

The therapy treatments

Before we start with the therapy protocols, I want to give you a description of the different types of natural therapies included and integrated in the biotherapy treatment protocols presented in the next chapter, which could be complementary or alternative in some cases to the conventional cures.

I'm also going to present a compendium of low dose (homeopathic) cytokines, hormones and growth factors which can be used and integrated in the treatments.

Phytotherapy or Herbalism

Phytotherapy or Herbalism is the therapeutic use of extracts from plants of natural origin as remedies. The herbal preparations are then standardized, which means that they are grown, harvested, and processed in a way which is designed to create a very reliable and stable dose of active ingredients.

Homeopathy

The theory of homeopathy was developed by the physician Samuel Hahnemann (1755–1843). Samuel Hahnemann developed the principle that a substance which will create the symptoms of a disease in a healthy person will actually cure the symptoms of the disease in a sick person. Hahnemann called this principle *"similia similibus curentur"* or "let like be cured by like". Homeopathy interprets diseases as caused by disturbances of the life force and sees these disturbances as manifesting as unique symptoms.

The homeopathic approach does not combat disease symptoms in the same way as one would in conventional medicine. Instead, homeopathic philosophy states that if the organism is brought back into balance, the symptoms of disease (imbalance) will resolve accordingly.

We immediately think about antiviral or anti-allergy vaccines. However, the use of vaccines is based on the 'principle of identity', in other words the cure is prepared using substances or materials which are the same as those which can cause the illness *(aequalia aequalibus)*, thus establishing a direct relationship between the pathogenic agent and the therapeutic agent (see **Prophylaxis against vaccinations side effects**). In homeopathy, this principle of identity gives way to the principle of similarity where the selected single remedy is based on the similarity to the *totality* of symptoms. **Hahnemann believed that by using remedies which would cause similar symptoms *as the totality of symptoms* of the original disease, the artificial symptoms would stimulate the vital force, causing it to neutralize and expel the original disease.**

This is accomplished by using various substances from the vegetal, mineral, and animal realm and using a process called 'dilution and dynamization' or 'potentization', whereby a substance is diluted with alcohol or distilled water and then vigorously shaken by 10 or 100 hard strikes against a hard base in a process called 'succussion'.

Although popular knowledge claims that Hahnemann discovered this method by striking the remedies on the Bible in order to empower them with the Holy Ghost, this process is now largely done in modern laboratories.

After Samuel Hahnemann, homeopathy was developed by many other physicians, among whom I'd like to mention James Tyler Kent (1849–1916), who integrated Hahnemann's ideas with Emanuel Swedenborg's (1688–1772) philosophy.

Kent believed that the overall picture of a disease was above all composed by emotional symptoms. He suggested that the true nature of a disease was not to be found by means of patho-logical anatomy, and that physical symptoms were just results of

a disease which started on a deeper level of emotions.
We can think of homeopathy as a unique therapy method
based on the original writings of Samuel Hahnemann and his
followers, but we can also use the aforementioned homeopathic processing principle called 'dilution and dynamization'
or 'potentization', and apply it with a modern and completely
different therapeutic view as we shall see with homotoxicology,
physiological regulating medicine and especially biotherapy.

Homotoxicology (complex homeopathy)

Homotoxicology uses complex homeopathic remedies with a
wide range of indications and is mainly prescribed according to
symptoms like in conventional medicine but with a completely
different aim: detoxification, immune modulation and organ
support. The German physician Hans-Heinrich Reckeweg
(1905–1985) developed homotoxicology as an integrative view of
allopathic medicine and homeopathy but the methodology of
homotoxicology differs from that of conventional medicine in
that the illness is seen as much more than the mere presence of
clinical symptoms. Homotoxicology is really the study of the
influence of homotoxins on the human organism. This
approach to illness sees disease as the result of the body's attempt
to heal itself by ridding itself of toxins which are either created
within the body as a result of cellular functions (endogenous) or
are taken in through the chemicals we are exposed to in our
environment (exogenous). In minor, self-limiting disorders, the
body detoxifies itself unaided, but in more serious situations,
treatment is needed. If the treatment used is able to eliminate the
toxins, then real healing can result. If the treatment suppresses
the toxins, as in conventional medicine, then they penetrate
deeper into the tissues and manifest after a latent period as a
more destructive disease. Homotoxicology applies Hering's Law
of Cure. According to the 19th century homeopath Constantine
Hering, healing progresses from the external to the internal or

deeper parts of the organism, and symptoms appear and disappear in the reverse of their original chronological order of appearance.

Homotoxicology definitely approaches the patient as a whole. It attempts to detoxify the body, to correct derailed immunological processes through immunomodulation, and to support cells and vital organs.

Physiological regulating medicine (PRM)

Physiological Regulating Medicine (PRM) represents an up-to-date integration of homeopathy, homotoxicology, Psycho-Neuro-Endocrine-Immunology (PNEI) and molecular biology. Physiological Regulating Medicine adds to classical homotoxicology a new therapeutic concept of restoring physiology through communicating molecules such as hormones, cytokines, interleukins, and growth factors prepared in homeopathic or low dose dilutions. These have the same physiological concentration (picograms to nanograms) as the molecules present in our organism which control and regulate organic functions under healthy conditions. We know that cytokines, hormones, growth factors and neuropeptides correctly diluted and potentized or dynamized (the homeopathic process) become active, through a mechanism of sensitization and activation of cellular receptors. We also know that the best way to correct a deficiency is to provide low doses of the same substance to stimulate its metabolism and physiologic production. **The result of the action of these homeopathic or low dose molecules is a physiological modulation of the cell's activity, when this is inhibited or disturbed by endogenous or exogenous stressors, and restoration of the capacities for cellular self-regulation which are indispensable for maintaining homeostasis.**

Micotherapy

Mushrooms are increasingly being evaluated in the West for their nutritional value and acceptability as well as their pharmacological properties. Increasingly, many are being viewed nutritionally as functional foods as well as a source of physiologically beneficial and non-invasive medicines, while others are distinctly non-edible but considered purely as a source of medicinally beneficial compounds. Some of the most recently isolated and identified compounds originating from the medicinal mushrooms have shown promising immunomodulatory, antitumor, cardiovascular, antiviral, antibacterial, antiparasitic, hepatoprotective and antidiabetic properties.

Certain medical mushrooms like reishi (*Ganoderma lucidum*), maitake (*Grifola frondosa*) and turkey tail (*Coriolus versicolor*) can be considered as multi-cytokine (interleukins, interferons and colony stimulating factors) inducers and have been shown to potentiate the organism's innate (non-specific) and acquired (specific) immune responses and activate many kinds of immune cells that are important for the maintenance of homeostasis, such as macrophages, monocytes, neutrophils, natural killer cells and dendritic cells.

Medicinal mushrooms have been studied extensively as supportive therapy for cancer, HIV, diabetes, candida, allergies and for antiviral activity.

We can find standard and low dose (homeopathic) mushrooms in various Biotherapy remedies and treatments.

Nutrition and dieting

Nothing in excess
Carving on the Temple of Apollo of ancient Greece

Nutrition and dieting is a vast and important subject related to maintaining good health, which I will not cover in this book as it is a subject of a book on its own. One important advice is to always try to find a balance or a compromise between the food that you like and the food that is good for you. In fact, although a diet rich in fresh fruit and vegetables is considerably healthier than a meat diet, it is important for example to consider particular foods which stimulate the 'feel good' brain neurotransmitters of dopamine and serotonin through those aliments containing the amino acids tyrosine, phenylalanine and tryptophan.

The 'feel good' brain molecules

Dopamine is the neurotransmitter needed for healthy assertiveness, sexual arousal and proper immune and autonomic nervous system function. Dopamine is also important for motivation and feeling pleasure and a sense of readiness to meet life's challenges.

Dopamine levels are depleted by stress, poor sleep, alcohol, caffeine and sugar.

Foods that increase dopamine levels include bananas, nuts and seeds, chicken, eggs, fish especially mackerel, salmon, striped bass, rainbow trout, tuna, and sardines, wheat germ, watermelon, beans, legumes and beets (betaine contained in beets acts as a stimulant for the production of **SAMe which is directly related to the production of dopamine and serotonin).** Dopamine is easily oxidized so it is advisable to eat plenty of fruit and vegetables whose antioxidants help protect dopamine-using neurons from free radical damage.

SAMe (S-adenosylmethionine) is a molecule which plays a role in the immune system, maintains cell membranes, and helps to produce and break down brain chemicals, such as serotonin, melatonin, and dopamine. It works with vitamin B12 and vitamin B6. Some research suggests that SAMe is more effective than placebos in treating mild-to-moderate depression. In addition, antidepressants tend to take 6–8 weeks to begin working, while SAMe seems to begin more quickly. Researchers aren't sure exactly how SAMe works to relieve depression, but they speculate it might increase the amount of serotonin and dopamine in the brain.

Serotonin is a neurotransmitter which plays an important role in regulating memory, learning, and blood pressure, as well as appetite and body temperature. Serotonin is the calming neurotransmitter important to the maintenance of a good mood. It promotes contentment and is responsible for normal sleep. Low serotonin levels produce insomnia and depression, aggressive behavior, increased sensitivity to pain, and are associated with obsessive-compulsive eating disorders.

Serotonin is synthesized from **tryptophan** in the presence of adequate vitamins B1, B3, B6, and folic acid, and is primarily found in the gastrointestinal tract (90%), where it regulates bowel movement, and in the central nervous system (CNS).

Foods rich in tryptophan include carbohydrates like pasta, turkey, ham, milk, brown rice, cottage cheese, meat, peanuts, and sesame seeds.

A natural source of tryptophan as a dietary supplement is the *Griffonia simplicifolia* plant (sold over the counter as 5-HTP). A seed extract of this plant taken daily naturally increases serotonin levels.

Another important neurotransmitter is **acetylcholine** which is the primary chemical carrier of thought and memory. It also plays a significant role in muscular coordination. A deficit in acetylcholine is directly related to memory decline and reduced cognitive capacity.

Acetylcholine's primary building block is choline which belongs to the B family of vitamins and is a fat-like substance that's necessary to metabolize fats. It is found in lecithin as phosphatidylcholine. Foods high in lecithin include egg yolks, wheat germ, soybeans, organ meats, and whole wheat products. Fish and algae are also important in the production of acetylcholine.

Vitamin C and B5 are needed for the brain to synthesize acetylcholine.

Deficiencies of acetylcholine result in mental and physical fatigue, inattention, ADD, ADHD, and loose skin.

Biotherapy

Biotherapy or Homeo Biotherapy is an innovative therapeutic approach which integrates homeopathy, homotoxicology, Physiological Regulating Medicine (PRM), micotherapy and nutrition and is the subject of the next chapter.

Chapter 13

General treatment protocols

The treatments and remedies presented in this chapter are very effective and mostly without side effects.

The general dose is 20 drops in a little water twice a day for the Phyto Biotherapy remedies and 15 to 20 drops twice a day for the Homeo Biotherapy complex remedies to be kept under the tongue for deep absorption before swallowing.

The therapy cycles should be of 2 weeks to 6 weeks depending on the specific condition, with short periods of rest (1 day to a week or longer).

The number that appears after the single remedies included in the Homeo Biotherapy treatments, in the complementary remedies, and in the low dose hormones and cytokines, refers to the homeopathic dilution of the remedy which can be expressed in the decimal scale (3X / 15X / 30X etc) or in the centesimal scale (3C / 4C / 6C / 15C etc).

The single remedies contained in the Phyto Bio remedies and the Homeo Biotherapy complex remedies can be chosen and combined according to the disease picture or your health practitioner's advice.

Both main and complementary treatments can also be combined to achieve a more complete effect on the PNEI system.

For children until the age of 12 the dose is usually 1 drop per year of the child's life, and the total day's doses should not exceed 20 drops.

The herbal remedies should be used only for children above the age of 6 in half the adult's dose.

In general, in choosing between the herbal therapy treatment and the homeopathic treatment you must bear in mind that the homeopathic treatments are gentler and with a deep and long-lasting effect as they work by stimulating or inhibiting organic functions with the therapeutic concept of restoring natural physiology.

The herbal or Phyto Bio remedies are slightly more aggressive and have a quicker effect, therefore can be used at the beginning of any treatment sometimes as alternatives to conventional drugs or if we want to see quicker results.

These advices are not to replace the advice of your doctor or professional health practitioners. Always seek professional help before starting a therapy.

Stress related conditions

Acute stress activates the sympathetic nervous system and the hypothalamic-pituitary-adrenal (HPA) axis, leading to heightened levels of catecholamines (epinephrine and norepinephrine) and steroid hormones like cortisol.

Many, if not most, of the diseases today can be linked to poor and stressful lifestyles and unresolved emotional issues. If we need to mention one psycho toxin above all else, it certainly needs to be the chronic stress hormone, **cortisol**. The physiological role of cortisol as a stress hormone is complex, but it seems its main role is to prevent the defense mechanism from overshooting in its response to prolonged stress. In the short-term, acute stress is mediated via the adrenergic system, but this cannot be sustained and if the stress is prolonged we see the characteristic detrimental effects of cortisol, which has an effect on so many levels.

The role of cortisol in cardiovascular disease and metabolic syndrome is becoming clearer. Central obesity is one of the metabolic actions of cortisol, and insulin resistance is a natural consequence. Cortisol also shares a receptor with the anabolic hormone testosterone in the muscle. If cortisol is constantly excreted at high levels over time, we see a displacement of testosterone, with resulting muscle atrophy and underperformance.

The effect of stress on the extracellular matrix is especially important, as cortisol plays a role in the natural degradation and repair process of the matrix. The phase when it goes down at midnight is a time where the slightly inflammatory state can clear up any diseased tissues in the matrix and also release toxins in the bloodstream. Insomnia and overwork will disturb this vital cycle, and keep cortisol up at night. This cleansing action cannot therefore take place and it is thus of extreme importance to restore the sleep cycle to allow this cleansing action.

We can also see that the corticotrophin-releasing hormone (CRH), another stress hormone, has receptors in the gut lining, thus causing an increase in the permeability of the gut with the resulting vicious cycles of allergy, intoxication, liver overload, and even systemic disease, which is triggered by the antigens leaking through the gut lining.

The importance of melatonin 'the long life hormone' in stress regulation

Melatonin is a derivative of serotonin. It is a neurohormone secreted by the pineal gland which is the most important neuroendocrine organ in the brain. Besides the regulation of circadian rhythms and sleep, the pineal gland hormone melatonin has been found to directly modulate catecholamine (epinephrine and norepinephrine) and cortisol levels.

The pineal gland translates an external signal (daily and seasonal variation in light and temperature) into a specific hormonal secretion which should regulate our endocrine functions. Alterations in circadian rhythms cause the onset of numerous pathologies like emotional problems (serious depression), immune deficiency, psychosomatic disorders, dermatological pathologies such as psoriasis and vitiligo, problems linked with appetite (bulimia, mental anorexia), sleep disorders, problems with puberty, initialization mechanisms for cancer etc.

Two thousand years ago, Herophilus spoke of the mysteries of the epiphysis (pineal gland), and Cartesio made it the seat of the soul.

Melatonin also controls the diurnal cycle of glucosteroids and inhibits hydrocortisone synthesis in the adrenal glands.

During stress, elevated amounts of hydrocortisone inhibit melatonin synthesis, thereby inhibiting the hydrocortisone 24-hour cycle with the consequence that hydrocortisone secretion becomes constantly elevated.

Chronic stress, typified by constantly elevated concentrations of hydrocortisone cause vascular damage, hypertension, type 2 diabetes and eventual organ failure.

Stress hormones affect memory processing, therefore **melatonin is a modulator of memory function**.

We can regard melatonin as a 'starter' which, depending on the gravity of the problem, has to regulate countless fragile mechanisms which ensure that our body is balanced.

Standard versus low dose (homeopathic) melatonin

In biological therapy, we need to work towards general regulation, both positive and negative; therefore we use an homeopathic dilution of the hormone. In cases where we want to induce a strong antioxidant effect or to induce sleep in people with severe insomnia as a substitute to sleeping pills, we can use a standard dose of 3 to 6 milligrams to be taken in the evening.

We can restore proper circadian cycles and lower stress levels using the Biotherapy treatments and the low dose melatonin combined with a detox and drainage treatment.

Phyto – Stress relief
Rhodiola rosea
Inositol
Uncaria tomentosa
Withania somnifera

Astragalus membranaceus

Magnesium

Impatiens

Elm

White Chestnut

Homeopathic treatment:

Bio-Stress relief

Interferon Gamma 4C

Nux vomica 4 / 9 / 15 / 30 / 200C

GCSF – granulocyte colony stimulating factor 4C

Argentum nitricum 9 / 15 / 30C

Gelsemium 12X

Adrenalinum 15–30C

Melatonin 4C

Glutathione 3X

Stomach suis 4C

Thalamus suis 4C

Dehydroepiandrosterone 6X

Centaury 1X

Agrimony 1X

Clematis 1X

Elm 1X

Impatiens 1X

Vervain 1X

Complementary remedies:

Citomix Guna: 3 granules twice a day

Anti age stress Guna: 3 granules three times a day

Nux vomica homaccord Heel: 15 drops twice a day

BDNF – Brain derived neurotrophic factor 4C: 15 drops twice a day

Coenzyme compositum Heel: One tablet per three times a day or
    1 ampoule three times a week

Ubiquinone compositum Heel: One tablet per three times a day or 1 ampoule three times a week

Melatonin: In insomnia 3 to 6 mg in the evening

Melatonin 4C: 15 drops twice in the evening

Griffonia simplifica seed extract (providing 5-HTP): 60 to 200 mg twice a day

Vitamin C: 2 grams a day

Vitamin D: 1000 IU a day

Inositol: 12 to 18 grams a day

Coenzyme Q-10 or ubiquinone (the most important antioxidant): 300 mg day

Magnesium: 500 mg a day

B complex Vitamin: 50 mg a day

Bach flowers: Centaury, Agrimony, Clematis, Elm, Impatiens, Vervain

Depression and anxiety

Depression is commonly divided in 4 types: Endogenous and exogenous depression, bipolar disorder and the Seasonal Affective Disorder (SAD).

In **endogenous depression** the underlining cause is more related to the body chemistry and/or to genetic factors therefore 'coming from within'.

Exogenous depression is primarily the result of upsetting and disappointing circumstances 'therefore coming from without'. In this case it tends to resolve as circumstances improve or as the individual adjusts to the circumstances.

Bipolar disorder also known as manic-depressive disorder manifests as alternating manic or irritable episodes, and major depressive episodes.

In most people with bipolar disorder, there is no clear cause for the manic or depressive episodes although the following may trigger a manic episode: life changes such as childbirth, medications such as antidepressants or steroids, long periods of sleeplessness and the use of drugs.

The manic phase may last from days to months. It can include the following symptoms: easily distracted, little need for sleep, poor judgment, poor temper control, reckless behavior and lack of self-control, binge eating, drinking, and/or drug use, spending sprees, very elevated mood, hyperactivity, increased energy, racing thoughts, talking a lot, very high self-esteem (false beliefs about self or abilities), very upset (agitated or irritated).

The depressed phase includes the following symptoms: daily low mood or sadness, difficulty concentrating, remembering, making decisions, eating problems, loss of appetite and weight loss, overeating and weight gain, fatigue or lack of energy, feeling worthless, hopeless or guilty, loss of pleasure in activities once enjoyed, loss of self-esteem, thoughts of death and suicide, trouble getting to sleep or sleeping too much, pulling away from friends or activities that were once enjoyed.

Sometimes the two phases overlap. Manic and depressive symptoms may occur together or quickly one after the other in what is called a mixed state.

Since there is a high risk of suicide with bipolar disorder, the person should not abuse alcohol or other recreational drugs, which can make the symptoms and suicide risk worse.

Since periods of depression and mania return in most patients even with treatment, the main goals of treatment are to prevent self-injury and suicide and make the episodes less frequent and severe.

Seasonal Affective Disorder (SAD) happens when a person's moods are unusually affected by periods of light and darkness. Symptoms usually build up slowly in the late autumn and winter months when they are predictably depressed.

In any depression and anxiety disorder it is preferable to reduce any sugar intake, and eliminate excitants like caffeine and related drinks.

In case you have been diagnosed with a bipolar disorder or an endogenous depression, it is important that you seek

professional advice before embarking in any therapy.

Physical exercise as mood therapy

Physical activity is strongly correlated with good mental health. Depression is related to low levels of serotonin and norepinephrine. Exercise increases concentrations of these neurotransmitters by stimulating the sympathetic nervous system. In addition, serotonin has a reciprocal relationship with the neurotrophin Brain Derived Neurotrophic Factor (BDNF). BDNF boosts serotonin production and serotonin stimulates BDNF expression. Since exercise also increases BDNF production directly, there is a reinforcement of the serotonin-BDNF loop, indicating exercise's significant potential as a mood-enhancer. **(For more information on BDNF and other neurotrophic factors see the section on geriatric conditions.)**

A recent study showed that physical exercise also stimulates the release of endorphins within approximately 30 minutes from the start of activity. These endorphins tend to minimize the discomfort of exercise and are even associated with a feeling of euphoria. Walking is especially good for the brain, because it increases blood circulation and the oxygen and glucose that reach the brain. Movement and exercise increase breathing and heart rate so that more blood flows to the brain, enhancing energy production and waste removal. Walking also improves learning ability, concentration, and abstract reasoning. Stroke risk was cut by 57% in people who walked as little as 20 minutes a day.

One of the best 'feel good' treatments is walking at an even and sustained pace for at least 30 minutes a day.

If you suffer from the exogenous depression and Seasonal Affective Disorder you can safely take the Biotherapy remedies and follow the treatments until an improvement of symptoms. In other cases you can combine the Biotherapy treatments with your standard medications according to your medical practitioner's advice.

Phyto – Anxious depression relief 1
Hypericum perforatum
Melissa officinalis
Humulus lupulus
Avena sativa
Mustard
Yerba Santa
Gorse
Wild rose
Willow
Heather
Agrimony

Phyto – Anxious depression relief 2
Griffonia simplifica seed extract (providing 5-HTP)
Melissa officinalis
Inositol
Rhodiola rosea
Mustard
Yerba Santa
Gorse
Wild rose
Willow
Heather
Agrimony

Homeopathic treatment:
Bio – Anxious depression relief
Serotonin 6X
5-Hydroxytryptophan 3X
Sepia 6 / 30C
Ignatia – 6 / 30 / 200C
Avena sativa 3X
Acidum phosphoricum 6 / 15X

Lycopodium 6C
Dopamine 6X
Pineal gland 6X
Zincum isovalerianicum 4X
Argentum nitricum 12X
Gelsemium 12X
Aurum metallicum 15 / 30X
Mustard 1X
Yerba Santa 1X
Gorse 1X
Wild rose 1X
Willow 1X
Heather 1X
Impatience 1X
Hypericum perforatum 2X

Complementary remedies:
Guna mood / Sepia comp: 15 drops twice a day
Guna awareness (support in bipolar disorders and autism): 15
    drops twice a day
Nervoheel / Ignatia Heel: 1 tablet three times a day
Dr. Reckeweg R14: 15 drops twice a day or 1 tablet three times a
    day
Tryptophan 6 D: 15 drops twice a day
Serotonin 6 D: 15 drops twice a day
Melatonin 4C: 15 drops twice in the evening
NGF – Nerve growth factor 4C: for more severe depressions 15
    drops twice a day
Neurotrophin 4 – 4C: 15 drops twice a day
Guna Tonic: 1 dose in the morning
Hypericum perforatum St. John's wort: 15 drops twice a day or
    300 mg AM and 300 mg PM
Griffonia simplifica seed extract (providing 5-HTP): 60 to 200 mg
    twice a day

SAMe-S-adenosyl-L-methionine: 200 to 800 mg a day on an
   empty stomach
B complex Vitamin: 50 mg
Vitamin D: 1000 IU a day
Inositol: 2 to 4 g twice daily or 3 times daily
Melissa officinalis: typically 1 to 2 capsules twice daily
Magnesium: 500 mg a day
Bach flowers: Mustard, Yerba Santa, Gorse, Wild rose, Willow,
   Heather, Impatience
**Note: In Bipolar disorders it is better to avoid SAMe, St.
John's wort (Hypericum perforatum), Ginkgo biloba, Ginseng
and 5-HTP.**

**In this case it is preferable a homeopathic treatment,
Inositol, Magnesium and Bach flowers in addition to your
prescription medication or according to your health practitioner's advice.**

St. John's wort (Hypericum perforatum) for depression and anxiety disorders

St. John's wort (*Hypericum perforatum)* owes its name to the fact
that it flowers at the time of the summer solstice around St.
John's day on 24th June. Having been administered as a remedy
by the Roman military doctor Proscurides as early as the 1st
century AD, it was mainly used for magic potions during the
Middle Ages. Historical information dating back to 400 BC tells
the story of hypericum and its medicinal and spiritual
evolution. The ancient Greeks and Romans noted that St. John's
wort was used for such things as snake or reptile bites, menstrual
cramping, gastrointestinal distress, ulcers, depression or melan-
choly, superficial wounds, or sciatica. First century Greek physicians, Galen and Dioscorides, recommended its use as a diuretic,
a wound healing herb and as a treatment for menstrual
disorders.

Paracelsus (1493–1541) was also concerned with St. John's

wort. He suggested that the bright, ray-like petals release their precious red liquid most efficiently when soaked in olive oil and left out in the sun for several days. This produces a thick, red liquid which could be then be applied externally on wounds, sprains, bruises and varicose veins.

In the Middle Ages the use of the herb extended into the spiritual or mystical realm as they believed the odor alone would drive off evil spirits, offering protection against the devil's temptations. This ancient belief that St. John's Wort conferred protection against evil spirits may have risen due to its use by traditional healers as a treatment for 'melancholia' or what was known at that time as 'troubled spirits'. It was assumed that when the mood of a person was down, sad or unsettled, this was the work of evil forces or demons.

However, in more recent times it has found its place mainly in the treatment of depression and anxiety disorders. Its action may be due to several chemicals, including hypericin, hyperforin, and flavonoids which stimulate the production of the 'feel good' brain chemicals serotonin, dopamine, and norepinephrine.

In fact there is good evidence that St. John's wort may reduce symptoms in people with mild-to-moderate depression. In many studies it seemed to work as well as selective serotonin reuptake inhibitors (SSRIs), a popular type of antidepressant.

St. John's wort can also be used to treat the following conditions, a few of which are related to depression.

- **Pre-menstrual syndrome (PMS):** Some studies suggest that St. John's wort may help relieve physical and emotional symptoms of PMS in some women, including cramps, irritability, food cravings, and breast tenderness.
- **Menopause:** Two studies suggest that St. John's wort helps improve mood and anxiety during menopause.
- **Seasonal affective disorder (SAD):** Used alone, St. John's wort has improved mood in people with SAD.

- **Eczema, wounds, minor burns, hemorrhoids:** St. John's wort has antibacterial properties and may also help fight inflammation. Applied topically to the skin, it may relieve symptoms associated with minor wounds and skin irritation.

The recommended dose should be of 300 mg (standardized to 0.3% hypericin extract), three times a day or 3 to 5 ml of mother tincture a day for long periods.

Note: St. John's wort can cause many interactions with prescription drugs. In most cases, St. John's wort makes the medication less effective. In few other cases, St. John's wort may make the effects of a medication stronger.

If you are using conventional medications, especially for mood disorders, you should not use St. John's wort without consulting a health practitioner.

Insomnia and sleeping problems:

Phyto – Sleep aid
Chamomilla recutita
Crataegus
Eschscholzia californica
Humulus lupulus
Tilia vulgaris
Melilotus
Avena sativa
Papaver rhoeas
Impatience
Vervain
White Chestnut
Rock Rose
Aspen

Bio – Sleep and anti-jet lag

Pineal gland suis 6X

Melatonin 3X

Serotonin 7C

Lavandula 1X

Crataegus 1X

Melilotus 1X

Melissa officinalis 3X

GABA 3X

Ignatia 4X

Avena sativa 3X

Chamomilla recutita 1X

Zincum isovalerianicum 4X

Coffea cruda 15X

Lithium gluconicum 4X

Tilia 1X

Impatience 1X

Vervain 1X

White Chestnut 1X

Rock Rose 1X

Aspen 1X

Complementary remedies:

Nervoheel / Ignatia Heel: 1 tablet three times a day

Dr. Reckeweg R14: 15 drops twice in the evening or 1 tablet three
times a day or during the night

Melatonin: 3 to 6 mg in the evening

Melatonin 4C: 15 drops twice in the evening

Anti age Reg Guna: 3 granules before sleep

Valeriana officinalis: standardized to contain 0.8% valerenic acid,
250 mg, twice daily or 2 at night.

Any herbal remedy containing: Chamomilla recutita, Crataegus,
Eschscholzia californica, Humulus lupulus, Tilia vulgaris,
Melilotus, Avena sativa

Magnesium: 500 mg a day

Griffonia simplifica seed extract (providing 5-HTP): 60 mg twice a day

Inositol: 2 to 4 g twice daily or 3 times daily

Bach flowers: Impatience, Vervain, White Chestnut, Rock Rose, Aspen

Detoxification and Drainage

(See Chapter 1 for a full explanation)

Matrix and Lymph system detoxification and support

Bio – Total detox

Interleukin 4 – 4C

Thuja occidentalis 6X

Urtica urens 3X

Fucus ves. 3X

Tyrosine 2X

Phenylalanine 2X

Histidine 2X

Lycopodium clavatum 6X

Chelidonium majus 3X

Nux moschata 3X

Carduus marianus 1X

Taraxacum officinale 4X

Cynara scolymus 4X

Aloe 2X

Nux vomica 3X / 6X / 12X

Sulfur 10X

Equisetum hyemale 3X

Hepar suis 6X

Duodenum suis 6X

Thymus suis 6X

Colon suis 6X

Vesica fellea suis 6X

Pancreas suis 6X

Cholesterinum 10X

Kidney suis 6X

Berberis 3X

Solidago virgaurea 1X

Urinary bladder suis 6X

Complementary remedies:

Guna Matrix: 15 drops in water twice a day

Guna-Lympho: 15 drops in water twice a day

Lymphomyosot: 15 drops in water twice a day

Galium Heel: 15 drops in water twice a day

Liver/Gallbladder detox

Phyto – Liver/Gallbladder detox

Pimpinella anisum

Silybum marianum

Cynara scolymus

Taraxacum officinale

Rheum officinale

Marrubium vulgare

Rosmarinus officinalis

Corylus Avellana

Curcuma longa Root

Cyclanthera pedata

Homeopathic treatment:

Bio – Liver/Gallbladder support

Taraxacum officinale 1X

Cynara scolymus 1X

Nux vomica 3X / 6X / 12X / 30X / 200X / 1000X

Lipase 6X

Transaminase 6X

Lycopodium clavatum 6X

Chelidonium majus 6X
Nux moschata 3X
Carduus marianus 1X
Hepar suis 6X
Pancreas suis 6X
Cholesterinum 10X
Vesica fellea suis 6X
Holly 1X
Beech 1X
Heather 1X
Pine 1X

Complementary remedies:
Heepel: 1 tablet three times a day
Nux vomica homaccord: 15 drops in water twice a day
Hepar compositum / Lycopodium comp Heel: 1 ampoule twice a
   week
Chelidonium homaccord: 15 drops twice a day
Anti2 Guna: 15 drops in water twice a day.
Anti age smog Guna: 3 granules three times a day
Dr. Reckeweg R7: 15 drops twice a day
Dr. Reckeweg R31: 15 drops twice a day

Kidney detox and support
Phyto – Kidney detox
Hieracium pilosella
Agropyrum repens
Asparagus officinalis
Juniperus communis
Solidago virgaurea

Homeopathic treatment:
Bio – Kidney detox and support
Kidney suis 6X

Berberis vulgaris 3X
Populus tremuloides 1X
Urtica urens 3X
Solidago virgaurea 1X
Plantago major 3X
Scrophularia nodosa 3X
Ureter suis 6X
Urinary bladder suis 6X
Betula alba 1X
Pilosella 1X
Equisetum hyemale 2X
Bacterium coli nosode 12X
Sarsaparilla 6X
Proteus 12X
Cantharis 6X

Complementary remedies:
Guna kidney/Pilosella comp: 15 drops in water twice a day
Berberis homaccord Heel: 15 drops in water twice a day
Populus compositum SR Heel: 15 drops in water twice a day
Solidago compositum Heel: 1 ampoule twice a week
Berberis compositum – Cosmochema: 15 drops in water twice a day
Dr. Reckeweg R27: 15 drops twice a day
Dr. Reckeweg R18: 15 drops twice a day

Bowels detox and support
Bio – Bowel regulation/ Hemorrhoids
Aloe 1X
Nux vomica 3X / 6X / 12X
Veratrum album 3X
Scatolum 6X
Lycopodium clavatum 6X
Rectum suis 6X

Taraxacum officinalis 1X
Carduus marianus 1X
Chelidonium majus 3X
Bryonia alba 6X
Colocynthis 12X
Paeonia 3X
Graphites 12X
Aesculus 6X

Complementary remedies:
Nux vomica homaccord Heel: 15 drops in water twice a day
Guna bowel: 15 drops in water twice a day
Guna hemorrhoids: 15 drops in water twice a day
Serotonin 6X: 15 drops in water twice a day
Dr. Reckeweg R37 (flatulence and constipation): 15 drops twice a day
Dr. Reckeweg R13 (hemorrhoids): 15 drops twice a day
Dr. Reckeweg R4 (diarrhea): 15 drops twice a day
Diarrheel / Tormentilla Heel (diarrhea): 1 tablet 3 times a day

Addictions (to be combined with the general detoxification treatment)
Guna addict 1 / metatox 1: 20 drops in water four times a day
Guna addict 2 / metatox 2: 20 drops in water four times a day
Nux vomica homaccord Heel: 20 drops in water twice a day
Griffonia simplifica seed extract (providing 5-HTP): 60 to 200 mg twice a day
Tryptophan 6X: 15 drops in water twice a day
Dr. Reckeweg R77 (nicotine addiction): 15 drops twice a day
Bach flowers: Beech, Crab Apple, Elm, Gorse, Gentian, Larch, Rock Water, Willow

Skin detoxification and support (to be combined with the general detoxification treatment)
Homeopathic treatment:
Bio – Skin
Skin tissue suis 6X
Coenzyme Q10 4X
Hepar sulfuris 30X
Arctium lappa 1X
Fumaria officinalis 3X
Urtica urens 3X
Alpha tocopherol 3X
Retinol 3X
Juglans 6X
Viola tricolor 6X
Thuja 6X
Sulfur iodatum 9X
Natrum muriaticum 30X
Lycopodium clavatum 6X
Nux vomica 6X
Graphites 12X
Streptococcus nosode 9C
Staphylococcus nosode 9C
Psorinum nosode 10X

Complementary remedies:
Apo reg Guna: 3 granules three times a day for dermatitis, dermatosis, acne
Anti age skin Guna: 3 granules three times a day
Psorinoheel: 15 drops twice a day (stimulation therapy for skin disorders and hepatic damage)
Cutis comp Heel: 1 ampoule three times a week for stimulation of the defensive system in cases of dermatitis, allergy, scleroderma, acne vulgaris
Dr. Reckeweg R21: 15 drops twice a day

Anti age face Guna: 3 granules three times a day

Anti age bronz Guna: (before and during sun exposure) 3 granules twice a day

FGF (Fibroblast Growth Factor) 4C: 15 drops twice a day in case of cicatrization difficulties

Vitamin E: 300 mg a day

Vitamin A: 3000 IU a day

Tamanu arnica cream Guna: Apply to affected skin in case of burns, scars, insect bites and for dry skin

Immune system support

The immune system is a system of biological structures and processes which protects the organism against any possible disease.

Disorders of the immune system can result in immuno-deficiencies, autoimmune diseases, chronic inflammatory diseases and especially cancer. Immunodeficiency occurs when the immune system is less active than normal, resulting in recurring and life-threatening infections and tumor proliferation.

We can divide the immune system into two main categories: the innate (non-specific) and adaptive (also known as acquired), although these distinctions are not mutually exclusive.

The **innate immune system** consists of cells and proteins that are always present and ready to mobilize and fight any antigen at the site of infection. An antigen may be a foreign substance from the environment such as chemicals, bacteria, viruses, or pollen or may also be formed within the body, as with bacterial toxins or tissue cells. Innate immunity refers to **non-specific** defense mechanisms that come into play immediately or within hours of an antigen's appearance in the body. These mechanisms include physical barriers such as skin, chemicals in the blood, and immune system cells that attack foreign cells in the body.

It is very effective but doesn't have a memory.

The **adaptive immune system**, on the other hand, is called into action against antigens that are able to evade or overcome innate immune defenses. Components of the adaptive immune system are normally silent and they come into play between 48 to 96 hours after an antigen's appearance in the body.

However, when activated, these components 'adapt' to the presence of infectious agents by activating, proliferating, and creating potent mechanisms for neutralizing and eliminating the antigen. There are two types of adaptive immune responses: **humoral immunity**, mediated by antibodies produced by B lymphocytes, and **cell-mediated immunity**, mediated by T lymphocytes. **Adaptive immunity includes a 'memory' that allows the organism to respond faster and more efficiently the next time it is exposed to the same antigen.**

Lymphocytes are an important type of white blood cell belonging to the adaptive immune system. There are B and T type lymphocytes. B lymphocytes become cells that produce antibodies. Antibodies attach to a specific antigen and make it easier for the immune cells to destroy the antigen. T lymphocytes attack antigens directly and help control the immune response. They also release chemicals, known as **cytokines**, which control the entire immune response.

To close, I'd like to mention the importance of **Natural killer cells** (or NK cells) and **cytotoxic T cells** or killer T cells in all infections and cancer proliferation. Natural killer cells are a type of cytotoxic lymphocyte critical to the innate and adaptive immune system. The role of Natural killer cells in adaptive immune responses is analogous to that of cytotoxic T cells. **Natural killer cells and cytotoxic T cells provide rapid responses to virally infected cells and respond to tumor formation, acting directly after infection.**

Using Biotherapy treatments we can regulate any area of the immune system and in particular the cell mediated immune responses through the activation or inhibition, if needed, of T cell lymphocytes, NK cells and macrophages. (See the use of

cytokines in the *cancer treatment* section.)

Viral and Bacteria infections:
Phyto – Total immune defense 1 – Also preventive
Echinacea angustifolia
Echinacea purpurea
Ginseng
Russian ginseng (Eleutherococcus senticosus)
Viscum album
Rosa canina
Malpighia punicifolia

Phyto – Total immune defense 2 – Also preventive
Ganoderma lucidum
Coriolus versicolor
Lentinus edodes
Cordyceps Sinensis
Rosa canina
Propolis
L-glutathione
Zinc

Homeopathic treatment:
Bio – Total immune defense – Also preventive
GCSF – granulocyte colony stimulating factor – 4 / 6C
Interferon gamma – 3C
Interleukin 2 – 4C
Interleukin 10 – 4C
Interleukin 4 – 4C
Ganoderma lucidum 1X
Coriolus versicolor 1X
Lentinus edodes 1X
Echinacea angustifolia 3X
Melatonin 4C

Asclepias Vincetoxicum 6X

Medulla ossis suis 4C

Thymus gland suis 4C

Lymphatic vessel suis 4C

Spleen suis 4C

Influenzinum nosode 9C

Streptococcus nosode 9C

Staphylococcus nosode 9C

Oscillococcinum Anas barbare (hepatis et cardus extractum) 9C

Complementary remedies:

Citomix Guna: 3 granules twice or three times a day – Also preventive

Dr. Reckeweg R87 Bacterial infections: 15 drops in water twice a day – Also preventive

Dr. Reckeweg R88: Viral infections – 15 drops in water twice a day – Also preventive

Guna Virus/NK Reg: 3 granules twice a day

Guna React/Macro Reg: 3 granules twice a day

Galium Heel: 20 drops in water twice a day – Also preventive

Engystol Heel: 1 tablet three times a day – Also preventive

Reishi mushroom (Ganoderma lucidum): 500 mg twice a day – Also preventive

Turkey Tail mushroom (Coriolus versicolor): 500 mg twice a day – Also preventive

Interferon Gamma 4C: 20 drops in water twice a day – Also preventive

Interleukin 2 – 4C: 20 drops in water twice a day – Also preventive

Interleukin 10 – 4C: 15 drops in water twice a day (anti-inflammatory to modulate all immune responses)

Anti-Interleukin 1: (anti-inflammatory to modulate all immune responses especially fever)

Anti age stress Guna: 3 granules twice or three times a day – Also preventive

Guna TF Papilloma: 1 capsule a day

Guna TF Candida: 1 capsule a day

Melatonin 4C: 15 drops twice in the evening – Also preventive

Vitamin C: 2 grams a day – Also preventive

Vitamin D: 1000 IU a day – Also preventive

Zinc: 15 mg a day

Seasonal Flu and Colds

Phyto – Flu and Cold relief – Also preventive

Harpagophytum procumbens

Salix alba

Echinacea angustifolia

Ginseng

Viscum album

Rosa canina

Malpighia punicifolia

Propolis

l-glutathione

Zinc

Homeopathic treatment:

Bio – Flu and Cold relief – Also preventive

Interleukin 2 – 4C

GCSF – granulocyte colony stimulating factor 4 / 6 / 15C

Interferon Gamma 4C

Interleukin 10 – 4C

Influenzinum nosode 9C

Oscillococcinum Anas barbare (hepatis et cardus extractum) 9C

Asclepias Vincetoxicum 6X

Echinacea angustifolia 3X

Apis mellifica 12X

Thymus gland suis 4C

Gelsemium 9X

Aconitum napellus 9X
Belladonna 9X
Allium cepa 6X
Lachesis 12X
Bryonia 9X
Cuprum 6X

Complementary remedies:
Citomix Guna: 3 granules twice a day – Also preventive
Guna flu: 1 tube 3 times a day for 2 days, or for prevention 1 tube
    every week from October until March (Northern Hemisphere)
Guna React/Macro Reg: 3 granules twice a day
Interferon Gamma 4C: 15 drops in water twice a day – Also
    preventive
Interleukin 10 – 4C: 15 drops in water twice a day (anti-inflam-
    matory to modulate the immune response)
Anti-Interleukin 1: (anti-inflammatory to modulate the immune
    response especially fever)
Interleukin 2 – 4C: 20 drops in water twice a day – Also
    preventive
Anti age stress Guna: 3 granules twice or three times a day – Also
    preventive
Vitamin C: 2 or 3 grams a day – Also preventive
Vitamin D: 1000 to 2000 IU a day – Also preventive
Zinc: 15 mg a day

Prophylaxis against vaccination side effects
Vaccines work by stimulating our immune system to produce antibodies (proteins produced by B lymphocytes of the adaptive immune system) and therefore protecting us against specific infections.

If, after vaccination, you come into contact with the disease itself, your immune system will recognize it and immediately produce the antibodies needed to fight it.

At first glance, this seems like a sound principle, BUT it only focuses on one aspect (antibodies produced by B lymphocytes) of the adaptive immune system (see Immune System Support for how the immune system works).

Research has revealed that vaccines can trigger immune system suppression by suppressing cell-mediated immunity (the part of the immune system which defends us against viruses and tumors) by depleting T lymphocytes.

Additives are also used in the production of vaccines and they may include preservatives and stabilizers to help the vaccine remain unchanged (e.g. albumin, phenols, and glycine), and adjuvants or enhancers to help the vaccine to be more effective.

Common substances found in vaccines include:

Aluminum gels or salts which are added as adjuvants to help the vaccine stimulate an earlier, more potent and more persistent immune response to the vaccine.

Antibiotics which are added to some vaccines to prevent the growth of bacteria during production and storage of the vaccine.

Egg protein is found in some vaccines like influenza and yellow fever vaccines, which are prepared using chicken eggs. People allergic or intolerant to eggs or egg products should avoid these vaccines.

Formaldehyde is used to inactivate bacterial products in some vaccines. It is also used to kill unwanted viruses and bacteria that might contaminate the vaccine during production. Most formaldehyde is removed from the vaccine before it is packaged.

Monosodium glutamate (MSG) and 2-phenoxyethanol, which are used as stabilizers in a few vaccines to help the vaccine remain unchanged when it is exposed to heat, light, acidity, or humidity.

Thimerosal is a **mercury-containing preservative** that is added to vials of vaccine that contain more than one dose to prevent contamination and growth of potentially harmful bacteria.

It is well known that substances like mercury and aluminum are in themselves immunosuppressing. Particularly, mercury causes changes in lymphocyte activity.

For example, a study from the New England Journal of Medicine of May 1996 revealed that the tetanus vaccine disables the immune system in HIV patients. The tetanus vaccination produced a drop in T cells in 10 of 13 patients, a classic sign of immune deficiency. HIV viral replication increased dramatically in response to tetanus vaccination.

Also the massive surge of antibodies created by the vaccine can cause the body to become hypersensitive and this is responsible for the increase in allergies and autoimmune diseases.

In fact, the word allergy is synonymous with sensitivity and inflammation. This is what vaccines do: they sensitize or render allergic an individual in the process of forcing him to develop antibodies to fight a disease threat. In other words, as part of the vaccine process the body will respond with temporary or long-standing inflammation.

Using Biotherapy treatments we can re-activate or stimulate cell mediated immune responses through the activation of T cell lymphocytes and NK cells. (See also the use of cytokines in the *cancer treatment* section).

Bio – Vaccination

(15 drops three times a day starting 1 day before vaccination and 15 drops twice a day for 10 days after the vaccination, **to be combined with the cell support antioxidant biotherapy)**

Interleukin 2 – 4C
Interleukin 12 – 4C
Interferon Gamma 4C
Melatonin 4C
Asclepias Vincetoxicum 6X
Medulla ossis suis 4C

Thymus gland suis 4C
Carduus Marianus 2X
Echinacea angustifolia 3X
Berberis Aquifolium 2X
Hepar Suis 4X
Ubiquinone 6X
Vaccinium Vitis 2X
DNA 6X
RNA 6X

Complementary remedies:
Before the vaccination:
Citomix: 10 granules the day of vaccination
NK Reg / Guna virus: 3 granules twice the day of vaccination
Reishi mushroom (Ganoderma lucidum): 500 mg twice a day
Turkey Tail mushroom (Coriolus versicolor): 500 mg twice a day
After the vaccination:
Citomix: 3 granules three times a day for a week
NK Reg / Guna virus: 3 granules twice a day for a week
Interleukin 12 – 4C: 15 drops twice a day for a week
Anti age cell Guna: 3 granules twice a day for a week
Reishi mushroom (Ganoderma lucidum): 500 mg twice a day
Turkey Tail mushroom (Coriolus versicolor): 500 mg twice a day

The role of Vitamin D in illness prevention

Vitamin D is a fat-soluble vitamin that is produced by our body when ultraviolet rays from sunlight strike the skin and trigger vitamin D synthesis. Season, time of day, length of day, cloud cover, smog, skin melanin content, and sunscreen are among the factors that affect UV radiation exposure and vitamin D synthesis. Complete cloud cover reduces UV energy by 50%; shade, including that produced by severe pollution, reduces it by 60%. UVB radiation does not penetrate glass, so exposure to sunshine indoors through a window does not produce vitamin D.

Sunscreens with a sun protection factor (SPF) of 8 or more appear to block vitamin D-producing UV rays. Individuals with limited sun exposure need to include good sources of vitamin D in their diet or take a supplement to achieve recommended levels of intake.

Vitamin D can be found in a small number of foods such as salmon, tuna, and mackerel and fish liver oils. Smaller amounts of vitamin D are also found in beef, liver, cheese, and egg yolks.

There are several forms of vitamin D, but the two forms that are more important for humans are vitamin D2 (ergocalciferol) and especially vitamin D3 (cholecalciferol).

Vitamin D promotes calcium absorption in the gut and maintains adequate serum calcium concentrations to enable normal mineralization of bones and, together with calcium, it also helps protect from osteoporosis. Without sufficient vitamin D bones can become thin and brittle and break easily.

Vitamin D is also an immune system regulator and stimulant. Laboratory and animal evidence as well as epidemiologic data suggest that vitamin D plays a role in the prevention of colon, prostate, and breast cancers. A growing body of research suggests that vitamin D plays a role in the prevention and treatment of seasonal affective disorder (SAD), influenza virus, type 1 and type 2 diabetes, hypertension, glucose intolerance and multiple sclerosis. Low levels of vitamin D also appear to be a risk factor for tuberculosis.

The suggested daily dose is 1000 to 2000 IU (*International Units*) **and most reports suggest a toxicity threshold of 10,000 IU a day.**

Autoimmunity

Autoimmunity can be the cause of a broad spectrum of illnesses known as autoimmune diseases. This happens because of misdirected immune responses targeting various organs and the body itself. Autoimmunity is present in everyone to some extent and is usually harmless, probably a universal phenomenon of vertebrate life. Autoimmune diseases are, thus, defined when the progression from benign autoimmunity to pathogenic autoimmunity occurs. This progression is determined by both genetic influences and environmental triggers.

Normally the immune system protects the body from harmful substances called antigens. Examples of antigens include bacteria, viruses, toxins, cancer cells, and blood or tissues from another person or species. In patients with an autoimmune disorder, the immune system can't tell the difference between healthy body tissue and antigens. The result is an immune response that destroys normal body tissues. This response is a hypersensitivity reaction similar to the response in allergic conditions; but in allergies, the immune system reacts to an outside substance whereas in autoimmune disorders the immune system reacts and targets normal body tissues or organs.

What causes the immune system to no longer tell the difference between healthy body tissues and antigens is unknown. One theory is that some microorganisms such as bacteria or viruses, drugs or environmental intoxicants in general may trigger some of these changes.

An autoimmune disorder may affect one or more organs and tissues. Organs and tissues affected by autoimmune disorders include: blood vessels, connective tissues, endocrine glands such as the thyroid or pancreas, joints, muscles, red blood cells and the skin.

Examples of autoimmune diseases include: Celiac disease, Multiple Sclerosis (MS), Diabetes Mellitus type 1 (IDDM), Systemic lupus Erythematosus (SLE), Sjögren's syndrome, Hashimoto's thyroiditis, Graves' disease, Crohn's disease, alopecia, psoriasis and rheumatoid arthritis (RA).

Using Biotherapy treatments for autoimmunity you can attempt to regulate immune reactions, monitoring with your medical doctor any improvement which might follow.

You should combine the general treatments with a full detox and drainage therapy and support the organs or tissues involved with a cell support-antioxidants therapy.

General homeopathic treatment for autoimmunity

Bio – Autoimmune
GCSF – granulocyte colony stimulating factor 6 / 15 / 30C
TGF1 beta 4C
Anti-Interleukin 1 alpha – 4C
Interleukin 10 – 4C
Interleukin 4 – 4C
Melatonin 4C
Gelsemium 18X
Holly 1X
Beech 1X
Crab Apple 1X

Complementary remedies:
Anti-Interleukin 1 alpha – 4C: 20 drops in water twice a day
Interleukin 10 – 4C: 20 drops in water twice a day
Melatonin 4C: 15 drops twice in the evening
Bach flowers: Holly, Beech, Crab Apple

Multiple Sclerosis

Multiple Sclerosis is an inflammatory autoimmune disease in which the body's immune system attacks and eats away the protective sheath (myelin) that covers the nerves. This interferes with the communication between the brain and the rest of the body, ultimately, resulting in deterioration of the nerves themselves, a process which is irreversible.

Symptoms vary widely, depending on the amount of damage and which nerves are affected. People with severe cases of multiple sclerosis may lose the ability to walk or speak. There's no cure at present for multiple sclerosis, however, treatments can help treat the attacks, modify the course of the disease and treat symptoms.

Using biotherapy treatments we can attempt to slow down and regulate the immune system reaction and reduce the inflammation.

Bio – Multiple Sclerosis support

Lathyrus sativus 6X

Phosphorous 12X

Acidum phosphoricum 18X

Magnesia phosphorica 9X

Gelsemium 12X

Anti-Interleukin 1 alpha – 4C

Interleukin 10 – 4C

Interferon Gamma 4C

TGF1 beta 4C

NGF 4C

Neurotrophin 3 – 4C

Neurotrophin 4 – 4C

Melatonin 4C

Crab Apple 1X

Agrimony 1X

Beech 1X

Complementary remedies:

Citomix Guna: 3 granules twice a day – Also preventive

Vitamin D: 1000 to 2000 IU a day – Also preventive

Anti-Interleukin 1 alpha – 4C: 15 drops in water twice a day

Interleukin 10 – 4C: 15 drops in water twice a day

Interleukin 4 – 4C: 15 drops in water twice a day

NGF – Nerve Growth Factor 4C: 20 drops in water twice a day

Guna cell: 15 drops in water twice a day

Melatonin 4C: 15 drops twice in the evening

Psoriasis

Psoriasis is an autoimmune disease that affects the skin. It occurs when the immune system mistakes the skin cells as a pathogen, and sends out faulty signals that speed up the growth cycle of skin cells. Psoriasis causes cells to build up rapidly on the surface of the skin, forming thick silvery scales and itchy, dry, red patches that are sometimes painful. Psoriasis patches can range from a few spots of dandruff-like scaling to major eruptions that cover large areas. Several types of psoriasis exist like plaque psoriasis, nail or scalp psoriasis and psoriatic arthritis. The cause of psoriasis is not fully understood, but it is believed to have a genetic component; environmental factors have been suggested as aggravating factors to psoriasis, including oxidative stress and withdrawal of systemic corticosteroid to name a few.

An autoimmune response is also involved in psoriasis where T cells lymphocytes which normally travel throughout the body to detect and fight off foreign substances, such as viruses or bacteria, start to attack healthy skin cells by mistake as if to heal a wound or to fight an infection. These changes result in an increased production of both healthy skin cells and more T cells and other white blood cells and this in turn causes an ongoing cycle in which new skin cells move to the outermost layer of skin too quickly (days rather than weeks).

Using biotherapy treatments we can attempt to slow down this cycle, reduce inflammation and regulate immune responses.

Bio – psoriasis
Anti-Interleukin 1 alpha – 4C
Interleukin 10 – 4C
Interleukin 4 – 4C
Melatonin 4C
Vitamin E 4X
Vitamin A 4X

Cutis suis 4C
Vena suis 4C
Collagen suis 4C
Ubiquinone 6X
Selenium 6X
Acidum fumaricum 10X
Natrium pyruvicum 10X
Holly 1X
Beech 1X
Crab Apple 1X

Complementary remedies:
Anti-Interleukin 1 alpha – 4C: 15 drops in water twice a day
Interleukin 10 – 4C: 15 drops in water twice a day
Interleukin 4 – 4C: 15 drops in water twice a day
Melatonin 4C: 15 drops twice in the evening
Stamibio Derm or Tamanu arnica cream Guna: apply cream
    topically twice a day
Anti age cut Guna: 3 granules two or three times a day
Anti age skin Guna: 3 granules two or three times a day
Guna cell: 15 drops in water twice a day
Acidum fumaricum-Injeel Heel: 1 ampoule twice a week

Seasonal Allergies
The immune system of people who are allergic reacts to different innocuous particles (called allergens) and treats them as invaders, releasing chemicals, including histamine, into the bloodstream to defend against them. It's the release of these chemicals that causes allergy symptoms.

Allergens can be found in a variety of sources, such as dust mite excretion, pollen from trees, grasses, flowers, pet dander or molds.

Seasonal allergies cause an inflammation of the mucous membranes that line the nasal passages and produce an array of symptoms, including eye irritation, sneezing, sinus pain (pressure or pain high up in the nose, around the eyes and at the front of the skull), congestion, shortness of breath and coughing.

Other allergic reactions involve irritation and inflammation (swelling) in various parts of the body. Food allergies are not as common as food sensitivity, but some foods such as peanuts, nuts, seafood and shellfish are the cause of serious allergies in many people.

The Biotherapy treatments will prove very effective and relieve you from most of the symptoms of seasonal allergies. The treatments should start at least 1 month before the allergic season and continue for the whole period.

In more severe cases it is advisable to do a desensitization treatment using homeopathic doses of the substances to which you are allergic in order to modify the allergic response.

Phyto – Allergy relief – Also preventive

Ribes nigrum
Rosa canina
MN – Manganese gluconate
Marrubium vulgaris
Luffa operculata
Galphimia glauca
Cardiospermum halicacabum
Aralia racemosa
Impatiens
Beech

Homeopathic treatment
Bio – Allergy relief – Also preventive

Interferon Gamma 4C
Interleukin 12 – 4C
Interleukin 10 – 4C
Asclepias Vincetoxicum 6X

Melatonin 4C

Adrenalin 9 – 15X

Histaminum 15 – 30X

Adrenalinum 9X – 15X

Manganese gluconate 3X

Sulfur 15X

Allium cepa 6X

Sabadilla 6X

Apis mellifica 12X

Galphimia glauca 6X

Glandula suprarenalis suis 6X

Luffa 6X

Natrum muriaticum 12X

Aralia racemosa 3X

Lobelia inflata 6X

Ribes nigrum 1X

Bio nasal spray

Euphorbium 6X

Luffa 6X

Sinusitis nosode 12X

Echinacea purpurea 3X

Allium cepa 6X

Pulsatilla 8X

Mucosa nasalis suis 6X

Sabadilla 6X

Apis mellifica 12X

Interferon Gamma 4C

Interleukin 12 – 4C

Anti-Interleukin 1 alpha – 4C

Histaminum 15 / 30X

Aralia racemosa 3X

Copper gluconate 4X

Ribes nigrum 3X

Complementary remedies:
Guna allergy prev: 15 drops twice a day as a preventive desensitization or any other products containing the same allergens to which you are allergic in homeopathic dilution. Start 1 month before the season.

Guna allergy treat: 15 drops three times a day during the whole season

Interferon Gamma 4C: 20 drops in water twice a day

Interleukin 12 – 4C: 20 drops in water twice a day

Interleukin 10 – 4C: 20 drops in water twice a day (anti-inflammatory)

Dr. Reckeweg R97 nasal spray: 3 to 5 times a day

Reishi mushroom (Ganoderma lucidum): 500 mg twice a day

Turkey Tail mushroom (Coriolus versicolor): 500 mg twice a day

Cancer treatment and prevention

The subject of cancer is a huge subject, and there are many complementary therapies on the market. The one that I propose works mainly with the PNEI system and is safe to use as a preventive or along with any other cancer therapy or conventional cure. **These curative treatments should be combined with the cellular and organ support therapies. Especially restoring the Krebs cycle and the cell mitochondrial function using the citric acid cycle catalysts** (see cell support and antioxidants), it is the mainstay in any cancer therapy. It's important to remember that any full detoxification and drainage therapy should be done only as cancer preventive at least twice a year but not during the cancer treatments whether they be conventional or alternative. In the latter case we should support the organs of detoxification which allow the body to detoxify at its own pace. Severely debilitated patients or patients who are in remission or post chemotherapy but still weakened should not undergo aggressive detoxification and drainage. Special care is also needed in patients with hormone-dependent cancers such as breast or prostate cancer, which may respond to endocrine-disrupting toxins released from the extracellular matrix. Detoxification and especially drainage should be extremely gradual in these patients. People that have completed cancer therapy and are officially in remission after subsequent check-ups should start a gradual detoxification and drainage, as these patients may have residual kidney and liver damage from aggressive chemotherapy. As a rule you should only start any complete detoxification and drainage therapies after a few weeks when the cancer standard or alternative cures have proven effective and you are in full remission.

In all tumor proliferation the importance of natural killer cells (or NK cells) and cytotoxic T lymphocytes cells (killer T cells) cannot be overemphasized. Lymphocytes are a type of white blood cell belonging to the adaptive immune system. T lymphocytes attack antigens directly and help control the immune response. They also release chemicals, known as **cytokines**, which control the entire immune response.

Cytotoxic T lymphocytes cells belong to the **adaptive immune system**, and express T-cell receptors that can recognize a specific antigen (a molecule capable of stimulating an immune response). **Their main role is to kill cancer cells, cells that are infected (particularly with viruses), or cells that are damaged in other ways.**

Natural killer cells are a type of cytotoxic lymphocyte of the **innate immune system**. The role natural killer cells play is analogous to that of cytotoxic T cells in the adaptive immune response. **NK cells provide rapid responses to virally infected cells acting directly after infection and respond to any tumor formation.**

Using Biotherapy treatments we can stimulate and regulate any area of the immune system and in particular the cell mediated immune responses through the activation of T cell

lymphocytes and NK cells so important in cancer prevention and therapy.

The important role of cytokines in both the innate and adaptive immune responses:

Cytokines are small messenger molecules released by cells that have a specific effect on the interactions between cells, on communications between cells and on the behavior of cells. We could say that cytokines are the hormones of the immune system.

Cytokines were officially recognized in 1979. Before 1979 immunologists believed that immune cells could not and did not secrete any chemical messengers. No one believed that the immune system was the cause of symptoms and signs of disease, because there was no known mechanism for the immune system to produce them. Thus, the discovery of cytokines created a revolution in immunology and medicine. Since that time, an enormous amount of research has been devoted to cytokines.

Cytokines are critical to the development and functioning of both the innate and adaptive immune response, although they are not limited to the immune system. They are often secreted by immune cells that have encountered a pathogen, thereby activating and recruiting further immune cells to increase the system's response to the pathogen. Cytokines are also involved in several developmental processes during embryo genesis.

Over-secretion of cytokines can trigger a dangerous syndrome known as a cytokine storm. Cytokine storms have potential to do significant damage to body tissues and organs. If a cytokine storm occurs in the lungs, for example, fluids and immune cells such as macrophages may accumulate and eventually block off the airways, potentially resulting in death. Cytokine storms were the main cause of death in the 1918 'Spanish Flu' pandemic, the 2003 SARS (caused by coronavirus) and the Avian Flu (A/H5N1) virus in 2008. Deaths were weighted more heavily towards people with a healthy immune system, due to its ability to produce stronger immune responses, with increasing cytokine levels.

Cytokines includes different types of molecules like interleukins, lymphokines and cell signal molecules, such as tumor necrosis factor (TNF) and the interferons, which trigger inflammation and respond to infections and cancer cells.

We can divide cytokines according to their biological role:

Growth factors which promote cell growth proliferation and differentiation; **Interleukins and lymphokines** which are capable of creating a communication network in the immune system and **chemokines and lymphokines** which are mainly involved in inflammation.

Unfortunately cytokines used by immunologists in conventional medicine and therefore in pharmacological doses have very strong and sometimes lethal side effects. **In biotherapy, on the other hand, we can safely use cytokines in low doses (homeopathic cytokines) and therefore without any side effects with the therapeutic concept of modulating and regulating immune responses and restoring natural physiology.** Low dose cytokines have the same physiological concentration (picograms to nanograms) as the molecules present in our organism and work through a mechanism of sensitization and activation of cellular receptors.

The result of the action of these homeopathic or low dose cytokines is a physiological modulation of the immune system cell's activity, and restoration of the capacity for cellular self-regulation.

List of the main homeopathic cytokines used in biotherapy and their therapeutic indications.

Interleukins:
Interleukin 1 – 4C: Used very rarely in biotherapy as an immune response starter and to induce a fever reaction.

Anti-Interleukin 1 – 4C: Regulates excessive production of pro-inflammatory Interleukin 1 and 6. **It is indicated in acute inflammatory conditions and fever, associated with the classic anti-inflammatory remedies. It is used to slow down articular cartilage degeneration. Also useful in some autoimmune diseases as rheumatoid arthritis, thyroiditis and multiple sclerosis.**

Interleukin 2 – 4C: Stimulation of T and B lymphocytes and NK cells. Regulation and stimulation of cell-mediated immune responses. **A very useful cytokine in immunodeficiency conditions such as AIDS, aging, recurrent viral infections, tumors and during chemotherapy.**

Interleukin 3 – 4C: IL-3 stimulates the hematopoietic stem cells into myeloid progenitor cells. **Indicated in hematopoietic disorders, neutropenia during and post chemotherapy, treatment of side effects of chemotherapy, radiotherapy and antiviral therapies, aplastic anemia.**

Interleukin 4 – 4C: Proliferation of B lymphocytes and mast cells. Synthesis of IgG and IgE antibodies. **Anti-inflammatory effect. Useful in most autoimmune diseases like diabetes type 1, rheumatoid arthritis and multiple sclerosis. It also has a pollutants detoxifying effect.**

Interleukin 7 – 4C: Proliferation of T lymphocytes especially cytotoxic T lymphocytes. It stimulates the hematopoietic stem cells into lymphoid progenitor cells. **Useful in immunodeficiency conditions such as AIDS, recurrent viral infections, tumors and during chemotherapy. Also used in wound repair.**

Interleukin 10 – 4C: Suppressant of most other cytokines. Regulation of the reactivity of the organism. **For regulating and modulating the immunotolerance processes and the inflammatory response. Useful in most autoimmune diseases and all chronic inflammatory conditions.**

Interleukin 11 – 4C: It is a pro-inflammatory cytokine. Increases platelet formation and is involved in bone formation. **It is indicated in bone healing with PTH (see low dose hormones), basic regulation during immunotherapy.**

Interleukin 12 – 4C: Stimulation of the NK cells and T lymphocytes. Stimulates cell mediated immunity. **Prevention of allergic manifestations, hypersensitivity and dermatitis. Useful in all immunodeficiency conditions such as AIDS and recurrent viral and bacterial infections. The most important cytokine with Interferon Gamma in cancer therapy.**

Interferon Alpha – 4C: Produced by infected cells. Activation of NK cells and T lymphocytes. **Antiviral activity. Useful in cancer therapy.**

Interferon Gamma – 4C: Activation of macrophages and NK cells. Reinforces T lymphocyte activity. **Antiviral and highly antibacterial activity especially during the onset of infections. Master cytokine in cancer therapy and preventive for cold and flu. Antiproliferative effects.**

Growth Factors:

TGF β 1 – Transforming Growth Factor beta 1 – 4C: Suppression of the function of the T and B lymphocytes and NK cells. **Involved in different stages of healing and connective tissue regeneration. Tendon, ligament and muscle repair.**

GCSF – Granulocyte Colony Stimulating Factor – 4C: Stimulates granulocytes (white blood cells). **Triggers the reactivity and raises the sensitivity of the immune system. Useful in the initial phase of all treatments and for chronic and autoimmune diseases. Very useful in neutropenia during and post chemotherapy.**

IGF 1 – Insulin-like Growth Factor 1 – 4C: For the growth and maintenance of nerve tissue. **Anti Age therapy. Involved in cartilage repair. Useful in metabolic syndrome and insulin resistance, obesity and high cholesterol levels.**

EGF – Epidermal Growth Factor – 4C: Stimulates epithelial cells, endothelial cells and fibroblasts. Stimulates angiogenesis **(contraindicated in cancer). Indicated in aesthetic applications to rejuvenate skin, repair sun damage, wound repair especially lacerations and burns. Gastric acidity.**

FGF – Fibroblast Growth Factor – 4C: Stimulates new growth of blood vessels, fibroblasts and endothelial cells. Stimulates angiogenesis **(contraindicated in cancer). Indicated in anti age therapy, metabolic syndrome and insulin resistance. Anti-inflammatory effect on muscle and bones.**

BDNF – Brain Derived Neurotrophic Factor – 4C: Neurotrophin with an effect on neurons growth and survival. **Useful in neurological damage, stress, depression, neurodegenerative**

diseases, Huntington's disease, Alzheimer's, Parkinson's, dementia, learning, memory and mood disorders. It is not indicated in case of migraines (see *Neurological and geriatric conditions*).

NGF – Nerve Growth Factor – 4C: Neurotrophin with an effect on growth, maintenance, and survival of certain target neurons of the nervous system. **Useful in neuralgic pain and neurological damage, memory, mood disorders and multiple sclerosis (see** *Neurological and geriatric conditions*).

Neurotrophin 3 – (NT3) – 4C: NT3 is a neurotrophic factor of the NGF (Nerve Growth Factor) family of neurotrophins. It helps to support the survival and differentiation of existing neurons, and encourages the growth and differentiation of new neurons and synapses. **Action similar to BDNF (see** *Neurological and geriatric conditions*).

Neurotrophin 4 – (NT4) – 4C: NT4 is a neurotrophic factor in the NGF (Nerve Growth Factor) family of neurotrophins. **Action similar to NT3 and BDNF (see** *Neurological and geriatric conditions*).

CNTF – Ciliary Neurotrophic Factor – 4C: CNTF is neurotrophin with an effect on the neurons where it promotes neurotransmitter synthesis. This protein is a potent survival factor for neurons and oligodendrocytes and may be relevant in reducing tissue destruction during inflammatory attacks. **Indicated in eyesight disorders, retinal degeneration, brain aging, appetite control.**

Cancer embryo therapy using low dose embryo preparations from zebrafish (Brachidanio rerio)

The aim of embryo therapy using low dose embryo homogenate preparations from zebrafish (*Brachidanio rerio*) is to

induce the activation of precise gene sites with a tumor suppressing action. Recent in vitro studies have proven that substances present in the embryo during cell differentiation are able to activate the **tumor suppressor protein p53.** The microenvironment of the embryo in oviparous appears to be the most effective in this kind of control. In fact this microenvironment is quite capable of leading the stem cells to a complete differentiation. In the course of cell differentiation the administration of known carcinogens can't induce any tumors in the embryo, probably because the genome control system is always active.

Recent studies show that the function of p53 in the embryo is to prevent malformations, to induce cell cycle arrest and apoptosis thereby preventing tumors. It can also activate DNA repair proteins when DNA has sustained damage and it regulates cell transcription especially during stress responses. Some authors have therefore defined p53 as "guardian of the baby" similar to the suppressor gene. Nevertheless, when embryonic stress is very severe and a large number of mutations are present, p53 can't repair DNA and causes the apoptosis of all cells (abortion). These processes take place also in tumor cells when p53 is activated. **In this sense tumor cells are similar to embryonic mutated cells.**

To conclude, we could say that the use of embryo homogenates from oviparous fish (*Brachidanio rerio*) in oncology is based on the observation that, during embryogenesis, exposure of the embryo to cancer causing substances leads to malformations, but never to cancer, which only occurs at a later stage of gestation, when the embryo has become a fetus. **Therefore it is possible to suggest low dose embryo therapy as a sort of physiological gene therapy with the aim to regulate the multiplication of cells and normalize physiological processes and to induce the activation of precise gene sites with a tumor suppressing action.**

References:

Biava, PM; Carluccio, A. Activation of anti-oncogene p53 produced by embryonic extracts in 'in vitro' tumor cells, Journal of Tumor Marker Oncology, 1997 vol. 12 n°4

Saunthararajah Y. et. al. p53-independent, normal stem cell sparing epigenetic differentiation therapy for myeloid and other malignancies. Semin Oncol 2012 Feb; 39(1)97-108

Zhao X., et. al. Recovery of recombinant zebrafish p53 protein from inclusion bodies and its binding activity to p53 mRNA in vitro. Protein Expr Purif 2010 aug; 72(2)262-266

Taira, N., Yoshida, K. Post-translational modifications of p53 tumor suppressor: determinants of its functional targets. Histol Histopathol 2012 Apr. 27(4)437-443

Homeopathic treatment
Bio – Cancer I and cancer prevention

GCSF 4C

Interferon Gamma 3C

Interferon Alpha 3C

Interleukin 12 – 4C

Interleukin 2 – 4C

Melatonin 4C

Aspergillus niger 8X

Candida albicans 8X

Ganoderma lucidum 1X

Coriolus versicolor 1X

Lentinus edodes 1X

Grifola frondosa 1X

Asclepias Vincetoxicum 6X

Medulla ossis suis 4C

Thymus gland suis 4C

Lymphatic vessel suis 4C

Thyroid gland suis 4C

Spleen suis 4C

Embryo rerio (*Brachidanio rerio*) homogenate 4X
Rock water 1X
Star of Bethlehem 1X

Bio – Cancer 2 and PNEI support

GCSF 4C
Interferon Gamma 3C
Interleukin 4 – 4C
Interleukin 12 – 4C
Interleukin 2 – 4C
Melatonin 4C
Somatostatin 6X
Medulla ossis suis 4C
Thymus gland suis 4C
Lymphatic vessel suis 4C
Thyroid gland suis 4C
Spleen suis 4C
Natrum oxalaceticum 6X
DL malic acid 6X
Viscum album 1X
Colchicum autumnale 5X
Conium maculatum 3X
Galium aparine 3X
Sempervivum tectoreum 4X
cAMP (cyclic adenosine monophosphate) 6X
Embryo rerio (*Brachidanio rerio*) homogenate 4X

Complementary remedies:
Guna Rerio (*Brachidanio rerio*) homogenate 4X: 30 drops in water
    twice or three times a day – Also preventive 20 drops twice a
    day for 6 weeks twice a year
Interferon Gamma 4C: 20 drops in water twice a day
Interferon Alpha 4C: 20 drops in water twice a day
Interleukin 12 – 4C: 20 drops in water twice a day

Melatonin: 2 to 6 mg in the evening to induce a strong antioxidant effect during chemotherapy

Melatonin 4C: 20 drops in water twice a day – Also preventive

Somatostatin 6X: 20 drops in water twice a day

Interleukin 2 – 4C: 20 drops in water twice a day

Galium Heel: 20 drops in water twice a day – Also preventive

Guna Virus/NK Reg: 3 granules twice a day – Also preventive

Reishi mushroom (Ganoderma lucidum): 500 mg twice a day – Also preventive

Turkey Tail mushroom (Coriolus versicolor): 500 mg twice a day – Also preventive

Guna TF Papilloma: 1 capsule a day – Also preventive

Guna TF Candida: 1 capsule a day – Also preventive

Vitamin C: 2 or 3 grams a day

Vitamin D: 1000 to 2000 IU a day – Also preventive

Guna Basic: 1 packet 3 days in a row, then 2 X week – Also preventive

Anti age stress Guna: 3 granules three times a day

During and after chemo and radiotherapy:

GCSF – granulocyte colony stimulating factor 4C: 15 drops in water twice a day

Interleukin 3 – 4C: 15 drops in water twice a day

Guna cell: 15 drops twice or three times a day

Coenzyme compositum Heel: One tablet per three times a day or 1 ampoule three times a week

Ubiquinone compositum Heel: One tablet per three times a day or 1 ampoule three times a week

Anti age stress Guna: 3 granules three times a day

Coenzyme Q-10 or ubiquinone: 300 mg day

HIV

HIV infects cells of the immune system and the central nervous system. One of the main type of cells that HIV infects is the T helper lymphocyte (Th lymphocytes) also called CD4 + Th-cell (CD4 is the protein expressed on their surface). These cells play a crucial role in the immune system, by coordinating the actions of other immune system cells. **A large reduction in the number of T helper cells seriously weakens the immune system.**

As we have seen, there are two major branches of the immune system, one which works through antibodies, produced by B-cells and plasma cells, and the other that works through direct cellular action and which relies heavily on CD4+ Th-cells. The first is called antibody-mediated or humoral immunity, and the second is called cell-mediated immunity. **It is the cell-mediated arm of the immune system that is found to be profoundly suppressed in people diagnosed with AIDS.**

AIDS is diagnosed when any condition of increasingly severe opportunistic infections and cancer is diagnosed and/or the CD4 count is less than 200 cells/mm3 with a percentage less than 15%.

We must also bear in mind that not only HIV causes a low CD4+ T-cell count but there is evidence that a multitude of viruses, parasites, bacteria infections, injected drugs and severe injuries interfere with the ability of CD4+ T-cells to proliferate.

You can safely add the Biotherapy treatments to your standard HIV medications, monitoring any signs of improvement of immune cells count especially the T helper lymphocyte (CD4).

Bio – HIV support

GCSF – granulocyte colony stimulating factor 4C
Interferon Gamma 3C
Interferon Alpha 3C
Interleukin 2 – 4C
Interleukin 7 – 4C
Interleukin 12 – 4C
Ganoderma lucidum 1X
Coriolus versicolor 1X

Lentinus edodes 1X

Echinacea angustifolia 3X

Pineal gland suis 6X

Melatonin 4C

Ginseng 1X

Asclepias Vincetoxicum 6X

Medulla ossis suis 4C

Thymus gland suis 4C

Lymphatic vessel suis 4C

Spleen suis 4C

Influenzinum nosode 9C

Streptococcus nosode 9C

Staphylococcus nosode 9C

Complementary remedies:
Interferon Gamma 4C: 20 drops in water twice a day
Interferon Alpha 4C: 20 drops in water twice a day
Interleukin 12 – 4C: 20 drops in water twice a day
Interleukin 7 – 4C: 20 drops in water twice a day
Melatonin 4C: 20 drops in water twice a day
Galium Heel: 20 drops in water twice a day
Guna Virus / NK Reg: 3 granules twice a day
T 4 reg Guna: 3 granules twice a day
Anti age stress Guna: 3 granules three times a day
Reishi mushroom (Ganoderma lucidum): 500 mg twice a day
Turkey Tail mushroom (Coriolus versicolor): 500 mg twice a day
Coenzyme compositum Heel: One tablet per three times a day or
    1 ampoule three times a week
Ubiquinone compositum Heel: One tablet per three times a day
    or 1 ampoule three times a week
Anti age stress Guna: 3 granules three times a day
Vitamin C: 2 or 3 grams a day
Vitamin D: 1000 to 2000 IU a day

Mycoses or Fungal infections

Fungal infections or mycoses cause a wide range of diseases. Mycoses range in extent from superficial infections involving the outer layer of the skin to disseminated infections involving the brain, heart, lungs, liver, spleen and kidneys.

There are over 100,000 different species of fungi, of which approximately 150 are known to be pathogenic to humans. **Fungi are organisms which live on decaying matter that are usually innocuous, but become pathogenic when the host becomes abnormally susceptible to infection.** For example, some yeast are present in the body in small quantities and are considered harmless; it is only when they get out of control and multiply excessively that problems are caused.

Pathogenic mycoses have been classified into four broad categories: superficial, cutaneous, subcutaneous and systemic.

Superficial mycoses are limited to the outermost layers of the skin and hair and usually elicit no inflammation.

Cutaneous mycoses may be classified as dermato-mycoses and dermatophytoses and are restricted to the keratinized layers of the skin, hair, and nails. **Unlike the superficial mycoses, immune responses are evoked, resulting in pathologic changes expressed in the deeper layers of the skin.** Dermatophytoses are caused by the agents of the *Epidermophyton, Microsporum, and Trichophyton* species. Dermatomycoses are cutaneous infections due to other fungi, the most common of which are the Candida species. A common cutaneous mycosis is *athlete's foot*, which usually affects men and children before puberty.

Subcutaneous mycoses enter the skin and cutaneous tissue usually in a traumatized area such as a wound; they usually remain localized, but can spread through the lymphatic system to other sites.

Systemic mycoses are believed to usually have a pulmonary inception, but can affect most areas of the body. They can be divided into primary and opportunistic systemic mycoses.

Primary systemic mycoses are able to establish infection in a normal host and usually gain access to the host via the respiratory tract; whereas opportunistic systemic mycoses require a compromised host in order to establish infection (e.g. cancer, organ transplantation, surgery, and AIDS). **Examples of opportunistic mycoses include candidiasis, cryptococcosis and aspergillosis.**

Systemic mycoses can cause a wide variety of health problems including digestive difficulties (diarrhea, bloating, discomfort, flatulence, constipation, etc.), skin problems (rashes, eczema, psoriasis, dry skin patches, intense itching, hives, open cut-like sores, etc.), bronchopulmonary disorders (asthma, breathing difficulties) fatigue, allergies, weight loss, fever, chills, malaise, depression, and chronic sinusitis; moreover some of them may be risk factors in developing autoimmune disorders.

Mycotic infections, though not normally fatal, are so under-diagnosed that an autopsy-based study found that in 22% of cases where the primary diagnosis was incorrect, the deceased had some type of fungal infection.

The range of patients at risk for invasive fungal infections continues to expand to encompass patients with acquired immunodeficiency conditions such as AIDS, alteration of normal flora by use of antibiotics, immunosuppressive therapy, and cancer treatments.

In most normal hosts or 'immunocompetent' people, systemic mycoses typically have a chronic course instead of being life threatening.

Keeping the skin clean and dry, as well as maintaining good hygiene, might help in preventing most fungal infections.

We must bear in mind that, as we have seen, according to homotoxicology and Biotherapy principles, disease is seen as the result of the body's attempt to heal itself by ridding itself of toxins which are either created within the body or are taken in through the chemicals we are exposed to in our environment. Therefore if our treatment suppresses the toxins (in this case the fungal infection) as in most conventional treatments, they go deeper into the tissues and manifest after a latent period as a more destructive and usually chronic disease.

We can safely use the Biotherapy treatments protocols as prevention and cure along with or without the standard conventional treatments for most fungal infections.

It also advisable to combine the specific Biotherapy treatments with a general detox and drainage and immune support therapy.

Homeopathic treatment

Bio – Myc – Also preventive
GCSF 4C
Interleukin 4 – 4C
Anti-Interleukin 1 – 4C
Interleukin 10 – 4C
Aspergillus niger 8X
Candida albicans 8X
Saccharomyces Apiculata 8X
Pityrosporum Orbiculare 8X
Penicillinum notatum 8X
Streptomyces griseus 8X
Natrum oxalaceticum 6X / 12X
Hydrocotyle asiatica 6X
Mercurius corrosivus 6X
Mucor mucedo 12X
Sulfur 6X
Melatonin 4C

Complementary remedies:
Mycox: 15 drops twice a day
Anti-Interleukin 1 – 4C: 15 drops in water twice a day

Interleukin 10 – 4C: 15 drops in water twice a day
Interleukin 4 – 4C: 15 drops in water twice a day
Anti age myc Guna: 3 granules twice a day
Eubioflor Guna: 15 drops twice a day
Guna TF candida: 1 capsule a day for 6 weeks
Psorinoheel Heel: (All skin mycoses) 15 drops twice a day

Cell support – Antioxidants

Antioxidants are substances that protect your cells against the effects of free radicals. Free radicals are molecules produced when your body breaks down food, or by environmental exposures such as tobacco, radiation and pollutants in general. One of the most common types of free radicals is oxygen free radicals. When an oxygen molecule ($O2$) becomes electrically charged it tries to steal electrons from other molecules, causing damage to the DNA of the other molecules. Over time, such damage may become irreversible and lead to disease including cancer. **Antioxidants interact with and stabilize free radicals and may prevent some of the damage free radicals might otherwise cause. Free radicals can damage cells, and may play a role in heart disease, hardening of the arteries, cancer and many other diseases.**

Antioxidants can be divided into six categories according to their potency level as follows:

1. Antioxidant systems like glutathione (GSH), catalase, super oxide dismutase (SOD) and peroxidase.
2. Antioxidants of mixed endogenous/food type (e.g. Coenzyme Q10, polyunsaturated fatty acids etc.).
3. Essential vitamins (e.g. Vitamin E, Vitamin C).
4. Carotenoid antioxidants. Carotenoids with molecules containing oxygen, such as lutein and zeaxanthin, are known as xanthophylls. The oxygen free carotenoids such as α-carotene, β-carotene and lycopene are known simply

as carotenes. β-Carotene, α-carotene and γ-carotene all have some vitamin A activity.

5. Flavonoid or bioflavonoids antioxidants sometimes referred to as vitamin P bioflavonoids are super-antioxidants found in many natural foods like red peppers, citrus fruits, tropical fruits, grape seed extract, strawberries, garlic, green tea etc.

Antioxidants can be found in many foods including fruits and vegetables, especially those with purple, blue, red, orange, and yellow hues, nuts, grains, and some meats, poultry and fish. **To get the biggest benefits from antioxidants, you must eat these foods raw or lightly steamed.**

Selenium is a mineral, not an antioxidant *per se*; however, it is a component of antioxidant enzymes. Plant foods like rice and wheat are the major dietary sources of selenium.

Energy metabolism and the citric acid cycle catalysts

The citric acid cycle also known as the Krebs cycle (after the German biochemist Hans Adolph Krebs who discovered it in 1937) is a key component of the metabolic pathway by which all cells that utilize oxygen as part of their respiration process generate energy. This cycle takes place inside the 'power plant' of the cells (the mitochondria) and provides the energy for the whole organism. The primary function of the mitochondria is to convert energy found in nutrient molecules and, through a long chain of reactions, store it in the form of molecular energy packets known as ATP (*Adenosine Triphosphate*). Since mitochondria require oxygen to carry out energy conversion, when oxygen is unavailable or the cycle is inhibited, the body shifts to a very inefficient way of producing energy through the path of glycolysis, which not only produces far less energy but also produces lactic acid as a by-product which is a cause of pain and inflammation in the muscles. It has been also known for decades that cancer cells perform glycolysis **only** to produce ATP. Different conditions like oxidative stress, illnesses, medicinal drugs, alcohol, food toxins and heavy metals such as mercury can also alter the cycle chemistry causing it to switch off energy production. A deficiency of one or more intermediate catalysts involved in the cycle and the consequent inhibition of normal energy production may cause a wide range of metabolic disturbances including fatigue, immune system dysfunction, dementia, depression, behavioral disturbances, attention deficiency, muscle weakness, heart diseases, diabetes, skin rashes, hair loss and eventually cancer. Impaired energy metabolism is also an indicator of Alzheimer's and Parkinson's disease. In terms of therapy, restoring the Krebs cycle and mitochondrial function is the basic starter point in any chronic disease and cancer therapy. Studies have shown that administering specific Krebs cycle amino acid precursors and catalysts to stimulate energy production significantly reduces the symptoms associated with low cell energy production.

Indications of low dose unitary Krebs cycle catalysts:

- Acidum citricum: neurological support, skeletal conditions, support calcium metabolism, digestive conditions.
- Acidum cis-aconitum: early signs of aging, hyper reactivity, hypersensitivity.
- Acidum succinicum: stress, debility after illness, neutropenia during and post chemotherapy.
- Acidum a-ketoglutaricum: functional nervous system support, stress, debility, general weakness.
- Acidum fumaricum: intoxication, liver and gall bladder conditions, food intolerance, metabolic syndrome.
- Acidum DL-malicum: glucose dysmetabolism, diabetes, hypo reactivity, chronic conditions, general detoxification, rheumatic conditions.

- Barium oxalosuccinic: general anti aging support, control of hormonal activity, impaired sight.
- Natrium oxalaceticum: vascular protection, immune system stimulation, susceptibility to infection.
- Natrium pyruvicum: slow metabolism, chronic conditions, food intoxication, skin conditions.

Bio Cell, Coenzyme compositum – Heel and Guna Cell contain all the low dose cell catalysts and elements to support and restore the Krebs cycle.

The biotherapy treatments offer a deep cellular detox and antioxidants support for a wide variety of conditions.

Phyto – Cell support – antioxidant

L-glutathione
Lycopene
Coenzyme Q10
Bilberry Extract
Beta Carotene
Alpha tocopherol
Alpha Lipoic Acid
Astaxanthin
Selenium
Zinc
Malpighia punicifolia

Homeopathic treatment
Bio – Cell support I (catalysts) – antioxidant

Methylglyoxal 10X
Acidum alpha-liponicum 3X
Acidum ascorbicum 3X
Acidum cis-aconiticum 3X
Acidum citricum 3X
Acidum fumaricum 3X

Acidum alpha-ketoglutaricum 3X

Acidum DL-malicum 3X

Acidum succinicum 3X

Barium oxalosuccinic 6X

Adenosinum triphosphoricum 10X

Thiaminum hydrochloricum 3X

Riboflavin 3X

Niacin 3X

Cobalamin 3X

Natrium diethyloxalaceticum 4X

Natrium pyruvicum 3X

Bio – Cell support 2 (quinones) – antioxidant

Methylglyoxal 10X

Coenzyme A 6X

Manganum phosphoricum 6X

Colchicum autumnale 6X

Conium maculatum 6X

Pulsatilla pratensis 6X

cAMP (cyclic adenosine monophosphate) 6X

Hepar sulfuris 6X

Sulfur 4X

para-Benzoquinone 10X

Ubichinon 8X

Naphthoquinone 8X

Anthrachinon 10X

Hydrochinon 8X

Selenium 2X

DNA 6X

RNA 6X

Complementary remedies:

Guna cell: 15 drops twice or three times a day

Coenzyme compositum Heel: One tablet three times a day or 1

ampoule three times a week

Ubiquinone compositum Heel: One tablet three times a day or 1 ampoule three times a week

Glyoxal compositum Heel: 1 ampoule a week for 6 weeks

Selenium Homaccord Heel: 15 drops twice or three times a day

Melatonin: 3 to 6 mg in the evening to induce a strong antioxidant effect

Melatonin 4C: 15 drops twice in the evening

Anti age stress Guna: 3 granules three times a day

Anti age smog Guna: 3 granules three times a day

Coenzyme Q-10 (ubiquinone): 300 mg day

Vitamin C: 2 or 3 grams a day

Vitamin E: 300 mg a day

Inflammation and pain

Inflammation is one of the first immune system responses to infection.

When tissue injury occurs, whether caused by trauma, viral or bacterial infection, heat, or any other occurrence, changes begin to occur in the injured tissue. Vasodilation (enlargement of the blood vessels), leakage of large quantities of fluid in the surrounding area, clotting of the fluid, and swelling of the cells are just a few of the immune system responses. The four classical signs of inflammation originally recorded by the Roman encyclopedist Celsus in the 1st century AD were *calor, dolor, rubor* and *tumor* equivalent to **heat, pain, redness and swelling.**

We must also understand that, especially during infections, acute inflammation is the first line of defense against the stressors. **By blocking inflammation, using anti-inflammatory drugs, we never allow complete healing and, instead, aggravate the situation in the long run by disrupting the capacities for cellular self-regulation which are indispensable for maintaining homeostasis.**

Especially when tissues do not heal correctly, not only is there chronic pain, but now inflammation, initially our friend, also becomes chronic and therefore our worst enemy.

So we should not suppress acute inflammatory processes but regulate them using the Biotherapy treatments before they become dangerous or chronic.

Phyto – Inflammation and pain relief

Acute phase: 15 drops every 15 min for max 2 hours then reduce to three times a day until remission – for chronic inflammation 20 drops twice a day for 4 to 6 weeks or longer

Harpagophytum procumbens

Salix alba

Equisetum arvense

Spirea ulmaria

Hypericum perforatum

Rock Rose

Homeopathic treatment
Bio – Inflammation and pain relief

Acute phase: 15 drops every 15 min for max 2 hours then reduce to three times a day until remission – chronic inflammation 20 drops twice a day for 4 to 6 weeks or longer

Anti-Interleukin 1 alpha – 4C

Interleukin 10 – 4C

TGF1 beta – 4C

Beta endorphin 6X

Aconitum napellus 9X

Belladonna 9X

Apis mellifica 9X

Bryonia alba 6X

Melatonin 4C

Arnica montana 3X / 6X

Calendula officinalis 1X

Mercurius solubilis 12X

Chamomilla recutita 1X
Hypericum perforatum 2X
Bellis perennis 3X
Rock Rose 1X
Star of Bethlehem 1X

Complementary remedies:
Acute inflammation: Acute phase: 15 drops every 15 min for max 2 hours then reduce to three times a day until remission
Traumeel /Arnica compositum
Guna flam: Acute phase
Anti-Interleukin 1 – 4C
Dr. Reckeweg R1
Harpagophytum procumbens
Beta endorphin 6X
Anti age dol Guna: 3 granules every 15 min then reduce to three times a day until remission
Chronic inflammation: 20 drops in water twice a day for 4 to 6 weeks or longer
Interleukin 10 – 4C
TGF Beta – 4C
Beta endorphin 6X
Harpagophytum procumbens (Devil's claw)
Anti-Interleukin 1 – 4C
Anti age dol Guna: 3 granules three times a day for 4 to 6 weeks or longer

Inflammation and Spasm
Homeopathic treatment

Bio – Spasm – Acute phase: 15 drops every 15 min for max 2 hours then reduce to three times a day until remission
Anti-Interleukin 1 alpha – 4C
Atropinum sulfuricum 6X
Berberis vulgaris 3X

Beta endorphin 4C
Magnesium phosphoricum 4X
Cobaltum metallicum 4X
Colocynthis 4X
Gelsemium 6X
Interleukin 10 – 4C
Passiflora incarnata 1X
Melatonin 4C
Chamomilla recutita 1X
Cuprum sulfuricum 6X
Ammonium bromatum 6X
Tilia tomentosa 1X

Complementary remedies:
Acute phase: 15 drops every 15 min for max 2 hours then reduce to three times a day until remission
Traumeel / Arnica compositum
Guna flam
Guna spasm
Anti-Interleukin 1 – 4C
Beta endorphin 6X
Spascupreel: 1 tablet every 10 minutes in acute phases for 2 hours then reduce to three times a day until remission
Chronic phase: 15 drops in water twice a day for 4 to 6 weeks or longer.
Interleukin 10 – 4C
Anti-Interleukin 1 – 4C
Melatonin 4C
Guna spasm
Magnesium: 200 to 500 mg for 4 to 6 weeks or longer

Skeletal system support (to be combined with the anti-inflammatory Biotherapy treatment)

Osteoporosis

Osteoporosis is a condition where the bones become thin and weak, and break easily. It frequently goes undiagnosed until a fracture occurs, as there are no warning signs. The spine, wrist and hips are particularly vulnerable to fracture.

Calcium from the diet and vitamin D, which is made by the body after exposure to the sun, are important factors for bone health. In fact the organism needs adequate supplies of vitamin D in order to absorb the calcium intake from the diet. Taking regular exercise is also very important in order to improve the strength of the bones. **Common risk factors for osteoporosis are long-term use of corticosteroid medications, smoking, heavy drinking, sedentary lifestyle, and estrogen deficiency following menopause in women.**

The biotherapy treatment should be followed for long periods with a week break every 6 weeks in order to improve symptoms and in some cases reverse the prognosis.

Phyto – Osteo

Harpagophytum procumbens
Urtica dioica
Salix alba
Glucosamine Hydrochloride
Magnesium
Methyl Sulfonyl Methane
Vitamin D
Zingiber officinalis

Homeopathic treatment
Bio – Osteo

Calcitonin 6X
PTH – Parathyroid hormone 6X

Glandula parathyroidea 10X / 30X

Abies pectinata 1X

Betula pubescens 1X

Equisetum arvense 3X

Silicea 6X

Vitamin D 1X

Calcarea phosphorica 12X

Calcarea fluorica 12X

Calcarea carbonica 12X

Ox suis 6X

Symphytum officinale 6X

Complementary remedies:

Calcitonin 6X: 15 drops twice a day

PTH – Parathyroid hormone 6X: 15 drops twice a day

Zeel Heel: 1 tablet three times a day or 15 drops twice a day

Osteobios Guna: 15 drops twice a day

Dr. Reckeweg R11: 15 drops twice a day

Vitamin D: 25 mcg a day or 1000 to 2000 IU a day

Sore Throat

Spray inside the throat 3 to 5 times a day.

Bio Throat spray

Interferon Gamma 4C

Belladonna 9X

Apis mellifica 9X

Calendula officinalis 1X

Mercurius solubilis 12X

Millefolium 3X

Asclepias Vincetoxicum 6X

Echinacea angustifolia 3X

Phytolacca americana 4X

Hypericum perforatum 2X

Propolis 1X

.Complementary remedies:
Guna throat spray: Spray inside the throat 3 to 5 times a day

Cough
1 dosage to be taken 3 to 5 times a day

Phyto – Cough syrup 150 ml
Thymus vulgaris
Juniperus communis
Malva sylvestris
Tilia tomentosa
Propolis
Papaver rhoeas
Petasites officinalis
Sambucus nigra
Echinacea angustifolia
Rosa canina
Eucalyptus globulus

Bio – Cough syrup 150 ml
Cuprum aceticum 8X
Drosera 1X
Sticta 3X
Bryonia 6X
Coccus cacti 6X
Sambucus nigra 1X
Echinacea angustifolia 1X
Ephedra vulgaris 2X
Thymus vulgaris 1X
Spongia tosta 12X
Eucalyptus globulus 2X
Antimonium tartaricum 8X
Rosa canina 1X
Rumex crispus 3X

Complementary remedies:
Guna cough / Homeotox noni: One dosage to be taken 3 to 5
times a day

Dr. Reckeweg R9: 15 drops twice a day

Migraine and Headaches (to be combined with a liver detoxification treatment)

A headache is a general name for pain or discomfort in the head, scalp, or neck. The most common types of headaches are likely to be caused by tight muscles in your shoulders, neck, scalp, and jaw and are called tension headaches.

Factors which might contribute to tension headaches are stress, depression, anxiety, bad posture, staying in one position for a long time, clenching one's jaw etc.

A migraine is a common type of headache that may occur with symptoms such as nausea, vomiting, or sensitivity to light. In many people, a throbbing pain is felt only on one side of the head.

Migraine attacks may be triggered by: alcohol, stress and anxiety, certain odors or perfumes, loud noises or bright lights, caffeine withdrawal, changes in hormone levels during a woman's menstrual cycle or with the use of birth control pills, changes in sleep patterns, exercise or other physical stress, missed meals, smoking or exposure to smoke. They can also be triggered by certain foods like: processed foods, fermented, pickled, or marinated foods, as well as foods that contain monosodium glutamate (MSG), baked foods, chocolate, nuts, peanut butter, and dairy products, foods containing tyramine, including red wine, aged cheese, smoked fish, chicken livers, figs, and certain beans, certain fruits like avocado, banana, or citrus fruit, meats containing nitrates like bacon, hot dogs, salami and cured meats.

It is believed that the attack begins in the brain, and involves nerve pathways and neurotransmitters like serotonin,

endorphins etc. The changes affect blood flow in the brain and surrounding tissues.

Although not all migraines are the same, typical symptoms include: moderate to severe pain, usually confined to one side of the head, but switching in successive migraines, pulsing and throbbing head pain, increasing pain during physical activity, inability to perform regular activities due to pain, nausea, vomiting, increased sensitivity to light and sound.

Some people who get migraines have a warning symptom called an aura before the actual headache begins. **An aura is a group of symptoms which may involve a temporary blind spot, blurred vision, eye pain, seeing stars or zigzag lines, tunnel vision etc.**

In many cases the recurrence and the severity of the attacks can be greatly reduced by using the Biotherapeutic treatments without the need of anti-inflammatory drugs (NSAID).

These specific treatments can be used at the onset of symptoms with a general dose of 15 drops every 15 min for 2 hours and then reducing the frequency until remission.

Phyto – Migraine – Headache relief

Tanacetum parthenium
Hypericum perforatum (St John's wort)
Harpagophytum procumbens (Devil's claw)
Salix alba
Crataegus
Chamomilla recutita
Melilotus officinalis
Cynara scolymus
Silybum marianum
Agrimony
Impatiens
Beech
Olive

Homeopathic treatment
Bio – Migraine – Headache relief

Cannabis indica 10X

Ignatia 4X

Gelsemium 12X

Arnica montana 3X

Iris versicolor 6X

Spigelia anthelmia 3X

Bryonia alba 3X

Melilotus officinalis 1X

Tabacum 9X

Sepia 9X

Beta endorphin 6X

Menyanthes trifoliata 6X

Tanacetum parthenium 3X

Glonoinum 12X

Serotonin 6X

Melatonin 4C

Impatiens 1X

Beech 1X

Olive 1X

Complementary remedies:

Serotonin 6X: 15 drops twice a day (especially for migraines)

Menyanthes compositum – Guna: 15 drops twice a day

Spigelon Heel: 1 tablet three times a day or 1 tablet every 10 minutes at the onset of symptoms

Spascupreel: 1 tablet every 10 minutes in acute phases

Traumeel / Arnica compositum: In acute phases 15 drops every 15 min then reducing the frequency until remission

Guna flam: 15 drops every 15 min for max 2 hours at the onset of symptoms then reducing the frequency until remission

Anti-Interleukin 1: 15 drops every 15 min for max 2 hours at the onset of symptoms then reducing the frequency until remission

Beta endorphin 6X: 15 drops every 15 min for max 2 hours at the onset of symptoms then reducing the frequency until remission

Chelidonium homaccord: 15 drops twice a day

Dr. Reckeweg R16: 15 drops twice a day

Dr. Reckeweg R81: 15 drops twice a day

Harpagophytum procumbens (Devil's claw): 15 drops every 15 min for max 2 hours at the onset of symptoms

Bach flowers: Impatiens, Beech, Olive, Rock Water

Vomit and nausea during migraine:

Vomitusheel / Apomorfin Heel: 15 drops every 15 min for max 2 hours at the onset of symptoms reducing the frequency until remission

Dr. Reckeweg R52: 15 drops every 15 min for max 2 hours at the onset of symptoms reducing the frequency until remission

Male and Female support (to be combined with cell support – antioxidant treatments)

Hormone replacement therapy versus low dose (homeopathic) hormone therapy

Hormone replacement therapy used to be a standard treatment for women with hot flashes and other menopause symptoms. It was also thought to have the long-term benefits for preventing heart disease and possibly dementia.

When a large clinical trial found that the treatment actually posed more health risks than benefits for one type of hormone therapy, particularly when given to older postmenopausal women, the use of hormone replacement therapy was dropped considerably.

In the largest clinical trial to date, a combination estrogen-progestin pill increased the risk of certain serious conditions, including: heart disease, stroke, blood clots and breast cancer.

Hormonal therapy is also one of the standard medical treatments for some types of cancer derived from hormonally responsive tissues, including the breast, prostate, endometrium and adrenal cortex.

In Biotherapy we use low dose (homeopathic) hormones always with the concept of restoring physiology by regulating the endocrine system through inhibition and stimulation feedbacks, without any side effect.

These specific treatments provide support for a wide variety of male and female conditions, such as lack of sexual desire, decreased sexual arousal, decreased sexual satisfaction, inability to maintain erection, discomfort during sex, vaginal dryness,

PMS, hormonal regulation etc.

Phyto – Male support

Selenium

Eleutherococcus senticosus

Magnesium

Chromium

Lycopene

Folic Acid

Pantothenic Acid

Impatience

Elm

Larch

Vine

Phyto – Female support

Salvia officinalis

Calendula officinalis

Verbena officinalis

Tilia tomentosa

Rubus ideaus

Sorbus domestica

Ribes nigrum

Folic Acid

Potassium

Inositol

Magnesium

Red Chestnut

Mimulus

Mustard

Homeopathic treatment
Bio – Male support

Damiana 4X

Orchitinum 6X

Dopamine 4X

Melatonin 4C

Serotonin 6X

Insulin-like growth factor 6X

Luteinizing hormone 6X

Lycopodium 12 / 30X

Selenium 3X

Conium 12X

Ubichinon 6X

Dehydroepiandrosterone 6X

Hypophysis 6X

Hypothalamus 6X

Testis suis 6X

Ginseng 3X

Eleutherococcus 3X

Ferrum phosphoricum 8X

Manganum phosphoricum 8X

Phosphorus 6X

Bio – Female support

Magnesium phosphoricum 10X

Sepia 12 / 30X
Dopamine 4X
Serotonin 6X
Oxytocin 6X
Insulin-like growth factor 6X
Melatonin 4C
Hypophysis 6X
Hypothalamus 6X
Moschus moschiferus 6X
Ignatia 6 /12 / 30X
Ovarium suis 6X
Placenta suis 6X
Corpus luteum suis 6X
Lilium tigrinum 4X
Lachesis 8X
Pulsatilla 18X
Folic acid 4X
Luteinizing hormone 6X
Follicle stimulating hormone 6X
Dehydroepiandrosterone 6X

Bio PMS

Melatonin 4C
Progesterone 6X
Beta estradiol 6X
Anti-Interleukin 1 alpha – 4C
Atropinum sulfuricum 6X
Beta endorphin 4C
Magnesium phosphoricum 12X
Cobaltum metallicum 4X
Colocynthis 4X
Passiflora incarnata 1X
Chamomilla recutita 1X
Cuprum sulfuricum 6X

Lilium tigrinum 6X
Lachesis mutus 6C
Hypophysis suis 6X
Ovarium sui 6X

Complementary remedies:
Male:
Guna Male / K2M (hormonal balance): 15 drops twice a day
Guna Mars (sexual related conditions, lack of sexual desire, decreased sexual arousal, decreased sexual satisfaction, inability to maintain erection): 1 tube contents to be dissolved in the mouth once a day preferably in the evening for 30 days
Selenium Homaccord: 15 drops twice a day
Phosphor Homaccord: 15 drops twice a day
Female:
Guna Fem / K2F (hormonal balance): 15 drops twice a day
Guna Venus (sexual related conditions, lack of sexual desire, decreased sexual satisfaction, discomfort during sex, vaginal dryness): 1 tube contents to be dissolved in the mouth once a day preferably in the evening for 30 days
Guna PMS: 15 drops twice a day
Hormeel (hormonal balance): 15 drops twice a day
Ovarium compositum Heel: 1 vial twice a week
Gynäcoheel: 15 drops twice a day
Dr. Reckeweg R10 (for menopause): 15 drops twice a day
Beta Estradiol 6X: (for menopause, hot flushes etc) 15 drops twice a day

Just like with cytokines, in Biotherapy we can safely use low dose (homeopathic) hormones without any side effects in order to regulate the endocrine system and restore homeostasis.

Low dose – homeopathic hormones and their main indications:

ACTH – Adrenocorticotropic hormone 6X: ACTH, also

known as corticotropin, is a trophic hormone produced and secreted by the anterior pituitary gland. It is an important component of the hypothalamic-pituitary-adrenal axis and is often produced in response to biological stress along with its precursor corticotropin-releasing hormone. It stimulates the production of corticosteroid hormones such as hydrocortisone, corticosterone, cortisol, aldosterone and the sex hormones. A deficiency of ACTH is a cause of secondary adrenal insufficiency and Addison's disease, and an excess can cause Cushing's syndrome. **Its main indications are: memory and learning deficiency, lack of motivation, asthenia, aging, chronic stress, inappetence, improvement of mental performance, visual alertness increase.**

β-**Endorphin 6X:** Beta endorphin is found in neurons of the hypothalamus, as well as the pituitary gland. It is used as an analgesic by the body to numb pain. The reason the pain dulls is because it binds to and activates opioid receptors. β-**endorphin has approximately 80 times the analgesic potency of morphine.** It is also believed to have a number of other benefits including slowing the growth of cancer cells, promoting a feeling of well-being and increasing relaxation. **Indicated in all pain therapies.**

Beta Estradiol 6X: Estradiol is a sex hormone. In females estradiol acts as a growth hormone for the tissue of the reproductive organs, supporting the lining of the vagina, the cervical glands, the endometrium, and the lining of the fallopian tubes. The development of secondary sex characteristics in women is driven by estrogens, and especially estradiol. **Its main indications are: estrogen deficiency, menopause, hot flushes, preservation of pregnancy, breast feeding maintenance and preparation for the menstrual cycle.**

Calcitonin 6X: Calcitonin is a hormone secreted by the thyroid gland. It helps to regulate calcium levels in the body inhibiting calcium reabsorption and opposing the effects of the parathyroid hormone. **It's highly indicated in osteoporosis and bone pain.**

Dopamine 6X: Dopamine is the neurotransmitter responsible for reward-driven learning, motivation, healthy assertiveness, sexual arousal and proper immune and autonomic nervous system functions. Several important diseases of the nervous system are associated with dysfunctions of the dopamine system among which we find: Parkinson's disease which is caused by loss of dopamine-secreting neurons in the substantia nigra, schizophrenia which has been shown to involve elevated levels of dopamine activity in the mesolimbic pathway, attention deficit hyperactivity disorder (ADHD) and restless legs syndrome (RLS) associated with decreased dopamine activity. **Indications for low dose dopamine are: mental stress, mood disorders and depression, decreased sexual arousal and lack of sexual desire, chronic fatigue syndrome and supporting treatment in Parkinson's disease.**

DHEA (Dehydroepiandrosterone) 6X: DHEA is an important steroid hormone produced by the adrenal glands, the gonads, and the brain. It functions predominantly as a metabolic intermediate in the biosynthesis of the androgen and estrogen sex steroids. It is an important regulator of the thyroid and pituitary glands and also has a variety of potential biological effects. DHEA is considered to buffer stress and the negative impact it can have on both mental and physical functions; it is a good stress barometer, because when stress levels go up, DHEA levels go down. Long-term stress can cause elevated cortisol levels and reduced DHEA levels with devastating effects on the immune system, with increased risk to infections, certain cancers, allergies and autoimmune diseases. Generally DHEA levels tend to decrease with age. High doses may cause aggressiveness, irritability, trouble sleeping, and the growth of body or facial hair on women. It also may stop menstruation and lower the levels of HDL cholesterol, which could raise the risk of heart disease. Regular exercise is known to increase DHEA production in the body. **Low dose DHEA is indicated in all stress related condi-**

tions, mood disorders and decreased sexual arousal and lack of sexual desire.

FSH (Follicle stimulating hormone) 6X: FSH regulates the development, growth, pubertal maturation, and reproductive processes of the body. FSH and luteinizing hormone (LH) act synergistically in reproduction by stimulating follicle maturation in women and spermatogenesis in males. **Indicated in ovulatory stimulation, female cycle disorders, female low libido.**

LH (Luteinizing hormone) 6X: LH stimulates development of the corpus luteum and estrogen production (with FSH) and progesterone production (with prolactin) in females. In males it stimulates testosterone production. **Indicated in male and female sterility, male low libido, female cycle disorders, recurrent abortion.**

Melatonin 4C: It is a neurohormone secreted by the pineal gland. It controls the neurohormonal system and normalizes the circadian rhythms. **Indicated in stress related conditions, insomnia and sleep disorders, jet lag, impotence, sterility, frigidity, mood disorders, cell proliferation, adjuvant in cancer therapy.** (See also **Stress related conditions**)

Oxytocin 6X: Oxytocin is a hormone that also acts as a neuro-transmitter in the brain. It is thought to be released during hugging, touching, and orgasm in both sexes. In the brain, oxytocin is involved in social recognition and bonding, romantic love, maternal behavior and may be involved in the formation of trust between people, and generosity. It plays a crucial part in enabling us to forge and strengthen our social relations. The inability to secrete oxytocin is linked to sociopathy, psychopathy, narcissism, inability to feel empathy and general manipula-tiveness. **Low dose oxytocin is indicated in: social phobia, decreased sexual satisfaction, female sexual conditions, support during delivery and support treatment for autism.**

PTH – Parathyroid hormone 6X: PTH is secreted by the parathyroid gland. It acts to increase the concentration of calcium in the blood. **It is indicated in bone repair processes, bone traumas, and bone formation, osteoporosis and low calcium levels.**

Progesterone 6X: It is a steroid hormone produced by the ovaries, the adrenal glands and during pregnancy in the placenta. It is involved in the female menstrual cycle; it supports gestation during pregnancy and embryogenesis. **It is indicated in menstrual cycle disorders, pre-menstrual syndrome (PMS), menstrual pain and pre-menopause.**

Serotonin 6X: Neurotransmitter derived from tryptophan. It is primarily found in the gastrointestinal (GI) tract where it regulates intestinal movements, and is synthesized in serotonergic neurons of the central nervous system (CNS). It is involved in the regulation of mood, appetite, and sleep. It also has some cognitive functions, including memory and learning. **Low dose serotonin is indicated in all mood disorders, depression, migraines, addictions and diet disorders.** (See also **Nutrition and dieting.**)

Somatostatin 6X: Somatostatin is an inhibitory hormone that regulates the endocrine system and affects neurotransmission and cell proliferation and inhibition of the release of numerous hormones. **Low dose somatostatin is indicated in: oncological diseases, cancer treatment, hyperthyroidism.**

Triiodothyronine (T3) 6X: T3 is a thyroid hormone produced by the follicular cells of the thyroid gland, which affects almost every physiological process in the body, including growth and development, body temperature, metabolism, and heart rate. T3 is activated by the thyroid-stimulating hormone (TSH), which is released from the pituitary gland. T3 increases the basal metabolic rate and therefore increases the body's oxygen and energy consumption. Because T4 is converted into T3 in target tissues, T3 is 3 to 5 times more active than T4.

Main indications for the use of this low dose hormone are: hypothyroidism with T3 deficiency and overweight tendency.

Thyroxine (T4) 6X: The thyroid hormone T4, just like T3, is produced by the thyroid gland and is regulated by TSH (**Thyroid-stimulating hormone**) released by the anterior pituitary gland. T4 is converted into T3 in target tissues, therefore thyroxine is believed to be a prohormone and a reservoir for the most active and main thyroid hormone T3.

Main indications for the use of this low dose hormone are: hypothyroidism with T4 deficiency, growth disorders, physical and neurasthenia, and overweight tendency. As T4 is converted into T3, this hormone should be the first choice in thyroid target therapies.

Thyroid-stimulating hormone – TSH 6X: TSH is produced by the anterior pituitary gland. It stimulates the thyroid gland to secrete the hormone thyroxine (T4) which is then converted into the active hormone triiodothyronine (T3), which stimulates and affects many physiological processes in the body including metabolism. About 80% of this conversion is in the liver and other organs, and 20% in the thyroid itself. **Main indications for the use of this low dose hormone are: thyroid stimulation, overweight tendency, obesity, short-term treatment for depression, neurasthenia, water retention and metabolic slowdown.**

Hypothyroidism

Hypothyroidism is a condition characterized by abnormally low thyroid hormone production. There are many disorders that result in hypothyroidism which may directly or indirectly involve the thyroid gland.

The thyroid gland is located at the front of the neck just below the larynx. It releases hormones that control metabolism, growth, development, and many cellular processes. **The thyroid itself is regulated by another gland located in the brain, called the pituitary gland or hypophysis.**

The pituitary gland releases the thyroid-stimulating hormone or TSH, which in turn sends a signal to the thyroid to release the two most important thyroid hormones which are thyroxine (T4) and triiodothyronine (T3). Once released from the thyroid gland into the blood, a large amount of T4 is converted into T3 – the active hormone that affects the metabolism of cells. If a disruption occurs at any of these levels it may result in a thyroid hormone deficiency or hypothyroidism.

Hypothyroidism is a very common condition. It is estimated that 3% to 5% of the population has some form of hypothyroidism. Iodine deficiency is the most common cause of hypothyroidism since the thyroid gland uses iodine mostly available from the diet in foods such as seafood, bread, and salt to produce the thyroid hormones T3 and T4. Iodine deficiency can also lead to a swelling of the thyroid gland called a goiter. More serious forms of hypothyroidism are Hashimoto's thyroiditis which is an autoimmune disease in which the body's immune system inappropriately attacks the thyroid tissue, and hypothyroidism due to pituitary disease, where for some reason the pituitary gland is unable to signal the thyroid and instruct it to produce thyroid hormones T4 and T3.

In areas of the world like Zaire, Ecuador, India, and Chile where there is an iodine deficiency in the diet, severe hypothyroidism can be seen in 5% to 15% of the population.

There are no herbs that contain thyroid hormones but there are some plants like seaweed, kelp and angelica sinensis, commonly known as 'dong quai' that have high concentrations of iodine.

The amino acid tyrosine taken in the morning has an indirect stimulation effect on the thyroid.

Selenium and zinc have a regulatory effect in all thyroid dysfunctions.

Homeopathic treatment
Bio – Hypothyroid

Spongia D3
Calcium jodatum D3
Thyroidinum D12
Hypophysis D12
Levothyroxinum D12
TSH 6X
T4 – 6X

Complementary remedies:

Lymphomyosot Heel: 15 drops twice a day

Strumeel: in goiter prophylaxis 15 drops twice a day or 1 tablet 3
    times a day

Dr. Reckeweg R19 – males: 15 drops twice a day

Dr. Reckeweg R20 – females: 15 drops twice a day

TSH 6X: 15 drops twice a day

T4 – 6X: 15 drops twice a day

T3 – 6X: 15 drops twice a day

Hyperthyroidism

Hyperthyroidism is a condition in which an overactive thyroid gland is producing an excessive amount of thyroid hormones that circulate in the blood. Some common causes of hyperthyroidism include: thyroiditis, an inflammation of the thyroid gland, excessive intake of iodine or excessive intake of thyroid hormones and the more severe Graves' disease.

Biotherapy treatment:
Bio – Hyperthyroid

Melatonin 4C
Somatostatin 6X
Ignatia 4X
Pineal gland suis 6X

Lavandula 1X
Melilotus 1X
Melissa officinalis 3X
GABA 4C
Avena sativa 3X
Chamomilla recutita 1X
Zincum isovalerianicum 4X
Impatience 1X
Vervain 1X
White Chestnut 1X

Complementary remedies:
Griffonia simplifica seed extract (providing 5-HTP): 50 mg a day
Dr. Reckeweg R19 – males: 15 drops twice a day
Dr. Reckeweg R20 – females: 15 drops twice a day
Melatonin 4C: 15 drops twice a day
Somatostatin 6X: 15 drops twice a day
Bach flowers: Impatience, Vervain, White Chestnut

Gastric conditions: gastritis, duodenitis, gastro-duodenitis
Phyto – Gastro

Ficus carica
Tilia tomentosa
Ribes nigrum
White Chestnut
Rock Water
Impatiens
Elm

Homeopathic treatment
Bio – Gastricum – soft lactose tablets

Abies nigra 6X
Anacardium orientale 6X
Antimonium crudum 6X

Arsenicum album 4X

Bismuthum subnitricum 6X

Carbo vegetabilis 6X

Nux vomica 4X

Argentum nitricum 6 / 12 / 30X

EGF – Epidermal growth factor 4C

Ipecacuanha 8X

Momordica balsamina 3X

Stomach suis 6X

Duodenum suis 6X

Petrolium rectificatum 6X

Robinia pseudoacacia 6X

Lachesis mutum 12X

Lycopodium clavatum 12X

Pulsatilla 6X

Chamomilla recutita 2X

Complementary remedies:

Guna stomach: 3 granules 3 times a day

Gastricumheel: 1 tablet 3 times a day

Duodenoheel / Ipeca Heel: 1 tablet 3 times a day

Dr. Reckeweg R5: 15 drops twice a day or 1 tablet 3 to 5 times a day

EGF – Epidermal growth factor 4C: 15 drops twice a day

Bach flowers: Impatience, Agrimony, Beech, Holly

Digestion support
Phyto – Digestion

Pimpinella anisum

Ananas sativus

Cynara scolymus Leaf

Curcuma longa Root

Taraxacum officinalis

Papain

Amylase
Bromelain
Protease
Lipase
Pomegranate Extract
Vaccinum myrtillus

Homeopathic treatment
Bio – Digestion

Hepar suis 6X
Pancreas suis 6X
Nux vomica 3 / 12 / 30X
Chelidonium majus 3X
Nux moschata 3X
Carduus marianus 1X
Taraxacum officinale 4X
Cynara scolymus 1X
Pimpinella anisum 1X
Vaccinum myrtillus 1X
Amylase 1X
Lipase 1X

Complementary remedies:
Guna digest: 15 drops twice a day
Nux vomica homaccord Heel: 15 drops twice a day
Chelidonium homaccord: 15 drops twice a day

Metabolic syndrome

Metabolic syndrome is the name of a group of risk factors that occur together and increase the risk of insulin resistance and type 2 diabetes, hypertension (high blood pressure), cholesterol abnormalities, an increased risk for clotting, coronary artery disease and stroke.

The most important risk factors for metabolic syndrome are:

Extra weight around the middle and upper parts of the body (central obesity). A high triglyceride level. (Triglycerides are a type of fat found in the blood.)

A low HDL cholesterol level which raises the risk for heart disease. (This is because HDL helps remove cholesterol from the arteries.)

Insulin resistance, where the body uses insulin less effectively than normal. Insulin is needed to help control the amount of sugar in the body. As a result, blood sugar and fat levels rise.

A high blood pressure, pushing the blood against the walls of the arteries as the heart pumps blood. If this pressure rises and stays high over time, it can damage the heart and can lead to plaque build-up.

Possible causes for metabolic syndrome are: aging, genetic reasons, hormonal changes and especially diet and lack of exercise.

It is advisable to combine the following treatments with the detoxification and drainage treatments.

Weight control treatment

Phyto – Weight control

L-Carnitine

L-Valine

L-Isoleucine

L-Lysine

L-Phenylalanine

L-Methionine

L-Tryptophan

Chromium

Impatiens

Centaury

Gentian

Homeopathic treatment

Bio – Weight control

Interleukin 10 – 4C

Urtica urens 3X

Tyrosine 2X

Phenylalanine 2X

Histidine 2X

Moschus 12C

Insulin-like growth factor 6X

Serotonin 6X

Dopamine 6X

Nux vomica 6 / 15X

Melatonin 4C

5-Hydroxytryptophan 3X

Argentum nitricum 12X

Hypothalamus Suis 9C

Sepia 6 / 30C

Ignatia 6 / 30C

Impatiens 1X

Centaury 1X

Gentian 1X

Complementary remedies:

Anti age dim Guna: 3 granules three times a day

Anti age fam Guna: 3 granules three times a day

Anti age diet Guna: 3 granules three times a day

SON formula Guna: 5 tablets a day (or as directed by your health
practitioner), to be swallowed with water during a meal

T4 6X: 15 drops twice a day

TSH 6X: 15 drops twice a day

Tryptophan 6X: 15 drops twice a day

Serotonin 6X: 15 drops twice a day

Dopamine 6X: 15 drops twice a day

Melatonin 4C: 15 drops twice a day

Diabetes support treatment

Bio – Diabetes

Adjuvant in type 1 (in addition to your insulin injection) and alone in type 2 insulin resistance conditions.

In both cases it is important to check and monitor insulin levels during the course of the treatment.

Pancreas suis 6X

Hepar suis 6X

Insulinum 4C

Syzygium jambolanum 3X

Secale cornutum 6X

Kreosotum 6X

Chromium metallicum 15X

Hypophysis suis 6X

Phlorizinum 6C

Lycopodium clavatum 4X

Hypothalamus suis 6X

Natrium sulfuricum 10X

Natrium choleinicum 6X

Melatonin 4C

Pineal gland suis 6X

Cobaltum gluconicum 6X

Complementary remedies:

For males – K2M DIA Guna: 15 drops twice a day

For females – K2F DIA Guna: 15 drops twice a day

Syzygium compositum Heel: 15 drops twice a day

Momordica compositum Heel: 1 ampoule twice a week

Nux vomica homaccord Heel: 15 drops twice a day

Dr. Reckeweg R40: 15 drops twice a day

Melatonin 4C: 15 drops twice a day

Galium Heel: 15 drops twice a day

Circulatory conditions

Phyto – Circulation

Sorbus domestica

Castanea vesca

Olea europea

Pine Bark extract

Vaccinium myrtillus

Lycopene

Coenzyme Q10

Homeopathic treatment

Bio – Circulation

Aesculus hippocastanum 1X

Secale cornutum 3X

Tabacum 10X

Artery suis 8X

Vein suis 8X

Apis mellifica 6X

Arnica montana 6X

Calcarea fluorica 8X

Hamamelis virginiana 2X

Lachesis mutus 8X

Viscum album 3X

Pulsatilla 8X

Mercurius solubilis 10X

Ferrum metallicum 10X

Belladonna 8X

Vaccinium Vitis 3X

Centella Asiatica 3X

Ananassa Sativa 3X

Complementary remedies:

Aesculus compositum Heel: 15 drops twice a day

Aesculus hippocastanum mother tincture: 30 drops twice a day

Anti Age Vein Guna: 3 granules three times a day

Dr. Reckeweg R67: 15 drops twice a day

Hypertension support treatment
Phyto – Hypertension

Allium sativum

Crataegus oxyacantha

Olea europea

Melilotus officinalis

Fraxinus excelsior

Beech

Impatience

Homeopathic treatment
Bio – Hypertension

Melilotus officinalis 1X

Crataegus 1X

Arnica 6X

Rauwolfia 3X

Aurum metallicum 15X

Passiflora 1X

Glonoinum 12X

Sulfur 12X

Baryta carbonica 12X

Adrenalinum 30X

Complementary remedies:

Melilotus homaccord Heel: 15 drops twice a day

Guna hypertension: 15 drops twice a day

Iper G Guna: 15 drops twice a day

Rauwolfia compositum Heel (constitutional high blood
    pressure): 1 ampoule three times a week

Crataegus mother tincture: 30 drops twice a day

Dr. Reckeweg R85: 15 drops twice a day

Melilotus officinalis mother tincture: 30 drops twice a day
Bach flowers: Beech, Impatience

Heart support treatment

Bio – Heart support
Arnica 3X
Cactus 3X
Spigelia 3X
Glonoinum 3X
Crataegus 1X
Strophantinum 9X
Cor suis 6X
Baryta carbonica 12X
Aconitum napellus 6X
Kalmia latifolia 4X
Kalium carbonicum 4X
Digitalis 6X
Valerian 2X

Complementary remedies:
Dr. Reckeweg R2 (cardiac arrhythmias, coronary circulatory disorders, angina pectoris): 10–15 drops 1 to 3 times a day; in acute cases: 10–15 drops 3 to 6 times a day
Dr. Reckeweg R3 (heart insufficiencies, myocardial weakness, heart diseases, degenerative processes of the myocardium, coronary insufficiencies): 10–15 drops 1 to 3 times a day; in acute cases: 10–15 drops 3 to 6 times a day
Cralonin Heel (geriatric heart, sequelae of myocardial damage, nervous cardiac disorders, piercing cardiac pain, and cardiac pain of other types): 15 to 20 drops three times a day
Cactus compositum Heel (coronary circulatory disorders, anginous symptoms, angina pectoris): 15–20 drops three times a day; in acute cases: 5–8 drops every 5 min
Cardiacum-Heel (anginous disorders, including those of

vertebral origin): in conditions where attacks occur 1 tablet every 5 minutes, otherwise 1 tablet three times a day

Glonoin-Homaccord Heel (tachycardia, throbbing palpitations extending to the neck, anginous disorders): 15 to 20 drops three times a day

Strophanthus compositum Heel (regulatory effect in coronary circulatory disorders, suspicion of myocardial infarction): 1 ampoule three times a week

Cor compositum Heel (stimulation of the defense system in cases of coronary circulation disorders, following myocardial infarction and cases of myocardial insufficiency): 1 ampoule three times a week

Neurological and geriatric conditions

The role of Neurotrophic Growth Factors (neurotrophins) in neurological and geriatric conditions

Growth factors such as neurotrophins that promote the survival of neurons are known as neurotrophic factors. Neurotrophic factors are secreted by target tissue and act by preventing the associated neuron from initiating programmed cell death – thus allowing the neurons to survive. **Neurotrophins regulate development, maintenance, and function of the nervous system.**

Neurotrophins also induce differentiation of progenitor cells to form new neurons.

Neurotrophins can be generally subdivided into four structurally related types: nerve growth factor (NGF), brain-derived neurotrophic factor (BDNF), neurotrophin-3 (NT-3) and neurotrophin-4 (NT-4).

The first one to be discovered by professors Rita Levi-Montalcini and Stanley Cohen was the **nerve growth factor (NGF)** in the 1950s; however, its discovery, along with the discovery of other neurotrophins, was not widely recognized until 1986.

Studies have shown that NGF seems to prevent or reduce neuronal degeneration in neurodegenerative diseases. It has also been shown to promote peripheral nerve regeneration. The expression of NGF is increased in inflammatory diseases where it suppresses inflammation. Dysregulation of NGF could also be involved in various psychiatric disorders, such as dementia, depression, schizophrenia, autism, anorexia nervosa, and bulimia nervosa. Dysregulation of NGF signaling has also been linked to Alzheimer's disease. **It also appears to promote myelin repair, therefore may be useful for the treatment of multiple sclerosis.**

According to some sources, Professor Levi-Montalcini's (now 103 years old) undiminished mental vigor is in part due to regular doses of nerve growth factor (NGF) in form of eye drops.

Brain-derived neurotrophic factor (BDNF) was the second neurotrophic factor to be discovered after nerve growth factor (NGF).

BDNF acts on certain neurons of the central nervous system and the peripheral nervous system, helping to support the survival of existing neurons, and encourage the growth and differentiation of new neurons and synapses. In the brain, it is active in the hippocampus, cortex, and basal forebrain – areas vital to learning, long-term memory, and higher thinking.

Exercise has been shown to increase the secretion of BDNF suggesting the potential increase of this neurotrophin after exercise although this seems to be cancelled out by exposure to air pollution.

Various studies have shown possible links between BDNF and conditions such as depression, schizophrenia, obsessive-compulsive disorder, Alzheimer's disease, Huntington's disease, dementia, as well as anorexia nervosa and bulimia nervosa.

Dr. John J. Ratey, a clinical professor of psychiatry at Harvard Medical School, in his book *SPARK: The Revolutionary New Science of Exercise and the Brain,* termed BDNF as "Miracle-Gro for the brain." Ratey explained that a massive amount of research has shown that **BDNF "nourishes neurons like a fertilizer."** When researchers sprinkle BDNF onto neurons in the lab, the cells spontaneously sprout new branches, producing the same structural growth required for learning.

Neurotrophin 3 (NT3): NT3 is a neurotrophic factor of the NGF (Nerve Growth Factor) family of neurotrophins. It was the third neurotrophic factor to be discovered after nerve growth factor (NGF) and BDNF (Brain Derived Neurotrophic Factor). **It helps to support the survival and differentiation of existing neurons, and encourages the growth and differentiation of new neurons and synapses.** (Action similar to BDNF.)

Neurotrophin 4 (NT4): NT4 is a neurotrophic factor in the NGF (Nerve Growth Factor) family of neurotrophins. **Action similar to NT3 and BDNF.**

Ciliary Neurotrophic Factor (CNTF): CNTF is a neurotrophin with an effect on the neurons where it promotes neurotransmitter synthesis. This protein is a potent survival factor for neurons and may be relevant in reducing tissue destruction during inflammatory attacks. **Its main indications are: eyesight disorders, retinal degeneration, brain aging and appetite control.**

Just like cytokines and hormones, in Biotherapy we can safely use the low dose neurotrophic factors without any side effects in order to regulate development, maintenance, and functions of the nervous system.

These treatments could be used as adjuvant treatments for memory loss, dementia and in Alzheimer's disease in addition to the specific complementary remedies.

Bio – Brain – memory

Aurum metallicum 6 / 12 / 30X

Lachesis mutus 12X

Melatonin 4C

Coenzyme Q10 – 3X
Selenium 3X
Manganese 4X
N-acetylcysteine 4X
Thyrotropin-releasing hormone (TRH) 3X
Brain derived neurotrophic factor (BDNF) 4C
Oxytocin 6X
Ciliary Neurotrophic Factor (CNTF) 4C
Neurotrophin 3 (NT3) 4C
Neurotrophin 4 (NT4) 4C
Cerebrum totalis suis 6X
Kalium phosphoricum 6X
Bufo rana 12X
Vanadium metallicum 6X
Ginkgo biloba 3X
Conium maculatum 4X
Thuja 6X
Ubiquinone 6X

Complementary remedies:
Cerebrum compositum Heel: 1 ampoule three times a week or 1
    tablet three times a day
Guna geriatrics: 15 drops twice a day
Guna awareness: 15 drops twice a day
Senectus Male: 15 drops twice a day
Senectus Female: 15 drops twice a day
Selenium Homaccord Heel: 15 drops twice or three times a day
Dr. Reckeweg R54: 15 drops twice a day
BDNF – Brain derived neurotrophic factor 4C: 15 drops twice a
    day
Neurotrophin 3 (NT3) 4C: 15 drops twice a day
Neurotrophin 4 (NT4) 4C: 15 drops twice a day
Oxytocin 6X: 15 drops twice a day
Insulin-like growth factor-1 (IGF) 4C: 15 drops twice a day

Guna brain: 1 tablet a day

Parkinson's disease:

Parkinson's disease is a disorder that affects nerve cells, or neurons, in a part of the brain that controls muscle movement. In Parkinson's, neurons that produce a chemical called dopamine die or do not work properly.

Parkinson's disease develops gradually, sometimes starting with a barely noticeable tremor in just one hand. But while tremor may be the most well-known sign of Parkinson's disease, the disorder also commonly causes stiffness or slowing of movement.

In the early stages of Parkinson's disease, the face may show little or no expression, or the arms may not swing when walking. Speech may become soft or slurred. Parkinson's disease symptoms worsen as the condition progresses over time.

As symptoms get worse, there may be trouble walking, talking or doing simple tasks. They may also be problems such as depression, sleep problems or trouble chewing, swallowing or speaking.

Biotherapy adjuvant treatments:

Extrabios 1 and Extrabios 2 Guna: 15 drops of each twice a day

Dopamine 6X: 15 drops twice a day

BDNF – Brain derived neurotrophic factor 4C: 15 drops twice a day

Neurotrophin 3 (NT3) 4C: 15 drops twice a day

Neurotrophin 4 (NT4) 4C: 15 drops twice a day

Cerebrum compositum Heel: 1 ampoule three times a week or 1 tablet three times a day

Guna awareness: 15 drops twice a day

Senectus F (female) or Senectus M (male) – Guna: 15 drops twice a day

Autism

Autism is a developmental disorder that appears in the first 3 years of life, and affects the brain's normal development of social and communication skills. It is characterized by impaired social interaction and communication, and by restricted and repetitive behavior.

Autism is a physical condition linked to abnormal biology and chemistry in the brain. The exact causes of these abnormalities remain unknown, but there is probably a combination of factors involved in autism.

Genetic factors seem to be important. Chromosomal abnormalities and other neurological problems are also more common in families with autism.

A number of other possible causes have been suspected like: diet, digestive tract changes, mercury poisoning, the body's inability to properly use vitamins and minerals, and vaccine sensitivity.

Environmental factors that have been claimed to contribute to or exacerbate autism include certain foods, infectious disease, heavy metals, solvents, diesel exhaust, pesticides, smoking, and prenatal stress.

Some studies suggest that the small amount of mercury that is a common preservative in most vaccines may trigger autism and attention deficit hyperactivity disorder (ADHD).

Biotherapy treatments may show some improvement of symptoms in most cases and are mostly without any side effects:

Homeopathic treatment (to be combined with the general detoxification and drainage treatment)

Bio – Autism complex
Mercurius solubilis 15/30X/200X
Mercurius corrosivus 15/30X/200X
Mercurius Cyanatus 15/30X/200X

Luesinum 30C
Hepar sulfuris 12X
Argentum nitricum 12X
Cerebrum suis 4C
Chelidonium majus 3X
Berberis vulgaris 3X
Passiflora incarnata 1X
Myristica sebifera 3X
Oxytocin 6X
Lycopodium 12X
Phosphorus 12X
Ribes nigrum 2X
Zincum isovalerianicum 6X
Niccolum metallicum 12X

Complementary remedies:
Oxytocin 6X: 15 drops twice a day
Magnesium: 200–400 mg
Vitamin B complex
Vitamin B6: 25 to 100 mg

Chapter 14

Concluding advice

Whatever method of treatment you follow don't forget to treat your mind, as body follows mind:

"As above so below."

The treatments and remedies presented in Part 2 are very effective and mostly without any side effects and can be combined with the visualizations and statements presented in Part 1.

Some minor conditions can be easily treated using the advices and natural treatments presented in this book. On the other hand, for chronic or more serious conditions and illnesses it is always advisable to consult a health practitioner or a doctor with knowledge in natural medicine before starting any therapy.

Even though it is true that homeopathic and low dose remedies are without side effects, if we choose the wrong treatment and persist in it we might aggravate our condition.

Sometimes during a treatment, especially at the beginning, we might notice an aggravation of symptoms, or new symptoms appearing in some other areas or tissues, but this is usually not a negative sign, but the first sign of healing. It happens generally when we do detoxification treatments and it usually resolves within days.

As we saw in homotoxicology, according to Constantine Hering, healing progresses from the external to the internal or deeper parts of the organism, and symptoms appear and disappear in the reverse of their original chronological order of appearance. This is sometimes observable and obvious, and sometimes not, therefore is always important to monitor changes with a health practitioner.

More information about Biotherapy can be found at this address:
http://www.homeobiotherapy.com
Additional Biotherapy research articles can be found at:
http://www.biopathica.co.uk/Article.htm
http://www.gunainc.com/pagina.php?mnu=5&id=33
For any general query regarding Biotherapy or to book an online consultation please contact:
max.corradi@homeobiotherapy.com
For any query regarding the production and distribution of the main Phyto and Homeo Biotherapy remedy formulations please contact:
info@homeobiotherapy.com
Twitter:
http://twitter.com/maxcorradi
Facebook:
http://www.facebook.com/pages/Homeobiotherapy/11860327
1487572
Biotherapy forum:
http://homeobiotherapy.creatingforum.com/

Appendix I

Main indications of low dose homeopathic hormones:
ACTH – Adrenocorticotropic hormone 6X: ACTH also known as corticotropin, is a trophic hormone produced and secreted by the anterior pituitary gland. It is an important component of the hypothalamic-pituitary-adrenal axis and is often produced in response to biological stress along with its precursor corticotropin-releasing hormone. It stimulates the production of corticosteroid hormones such as hydrocortisone, corticosterone, cortisol, aldosterone and the sex hormones. A deficiency of ACTH is a cause of secondary adrenal insufficiency and Addison's disease, and an excess can cause Cushing's syndrome. Its main indications are: memory and learning deficiency, lack of motivation, asthenia, aging, chronic stress, inappetence, improvement of mental performance, visual alertness increase.

β-Endorphin 6X: Beta endorphin is found in neurons of the hypothalamus, as well as the pituitary gland. It is used as an analgesic by the body to numb pain. The reason the pain dulls is because it binds to and activates opioid receptors. β-endorphin has approximately 80 times the analgesic potency of morphine. It is also believed to have a number of other benefits including slowing the growth of cancer cells, promoting a feeling of well-being and increasing relaxation. Indicated in all pain therapies.

Beta Estradiol 6X: Estradiol is a sex hormone. In females estradiol acts as a growth hormone for the tissue of the reproductive organs, supporting the lining of the vagina, the cervical glands, the endometrium, and the lining of the fallopian tubes. The development of secondary sex characteristics in women is driven by estrogens, and especially estradiol. Its main indications are: estrogen deficiency, menopause, hot flushes, preservation of pregnancy, breast feeding maintenance and preparation for the menstrual cycle.

Calcitonin 6X: Calcitonin is a hormone secreted by the thyroid gland. It helps to regulate calcium levels in the body inhibiting calcium reabsorption and opposing the effects of the parathyroid hormone. It's highly indicated in osteoporosis and bone pain.

Dopamine 6X: Dopamine is the neurotransmitter responsible for reward-driven learning, motivation, healthy assertiveness, sexual arousal and proper immune and autonomic nervous system functions. Several important diseases of the nervous system are associated with dysfunctions of the dopamine system among which we find: Parkinson's disease, which is caused by loss of dopamine-secreting neurons in the substantia nigra; schizophrenia, which has been shown to involve elevated levels of dopamine activity in the mesolimbic pathway; attention deficit hyperactivity disorder (ADHD); and restless legs syndrome (RLS) associated with decreased dopamine activity. Indications for low dose dopamine are: mental stress, mood disorders and depression, decreased sexual arousal and lack of sexual desire, chronic fatigue syndrome and supporting treatment in Parkinson's disease.

DHEA (Dehydroepiandrosterone) 6X: DHEA is an important steroid hormone produced by the adrenal glands, the gonads, and the brain. It functions predominantly as a metabolic intermediate in the biosynthesis of the androgen and estrogen sex steroids. It is an important regulator of the thyroid and pituitary glands and also has a variety of potential biological effects. DHEA is considered to buffer stress and the negative impact it can have on both mental and physical functions; it is a good stress barometer, because when stress levels go up, DHEA levels go down. Long-term stress can cause elevated cortisol levels and reduced DHEA levels with devastating effects on the immune system with increased risk to infections, certain cancers, allergies and autoimmune diseases. Generally DHEA levels tend to decrease with age. High doses may cause aggressiveness, irritability, trouble sleeping, and the growth of body or facial hair on women. It also may stop menstruation and lower the levels of HDL cholesterol, which could raise the risk of heart disease. Regular exercise is known to increase DHEA production in the body. Low dose DHEA is indicated in all stress related conditions, mood disorders and decreased sexual arousal and lack of sexual desire.

FSH (Follicle stimulating hormone) 6X: FSH regulates the development, growth, pubertal maturation, and reproductive processes of the body. FSH and luteinizing hormone (LH) act synergistically in reproduction by stimulating follicle maturation in women and spermatogenesis in males. Indicated in ovulatory stimulation, female cycle disorders, female low libido.

LH (Luteinizing hormone) 6X: LH stimulates development of the corpus luteum and estrogen production (with FSH) and progesterone production (with prolactin) in females. In males it stimulates testosterone production. Indicated in male and female sterility, male low libido, female cycle disorders, recurrent abortion.

Melatonin 4C: It is a neurohormone secreted by the pineal gland. It controls the neurohormonal system and normalizes the circadian rhythms. Indicated in stress related conditions, insomnia and sleep disorders, jet lag, impotence, sterility, frigidity, mood disorders, cell proliferation, adjuvant in cancer therapy. (See also **Stress related conditions**.)

Oxytocin 6X: Oxytocin is a hormone that also acts as a neurotransmitter in the brain. It is thought to be released during hugging, touching, and orgasm in both sexes. In the brain, oxytocin is involved in social recognition and bonding, romantic love, maternal behavior and may be involved in the formation of trust between people and generosity. It plays a crucial part in enabling us to forge and strengthen our social relations. The inability to secrete oxytocin is linked to sociopathy, psychopathy, narcissism, inability to feel empathy and general manipulativeness. Low dose oxytocin is indicated in: social phobia, decreased sexual satisfaction, female sexual conditions, support during delivery and support treatment for autism.

PTH – Parathyroid hormone 6X: PTH is secreted by the parathyroid gland. It acts to increase the concentration of calcium in the blood. It is indicated in bone repair processes, bone traumas, and bone formation, osteoporosis and low calcium levels.

Progesterone 6X: It is a steroid hormone produced by the ovaries, the adrenal glands and during pregnancy in the placenta. It is involved in the female menstrual cycle; it supports gestation during pregnancy and embryogenesis. It is indicated in menstrual cycle disorders, pre-menstrual syndrome (PMS), menstrual pain and pre-menopause.

Serotonin 6X: Neurotransmitter derived from tryptophan. It is primarily found in the gastrointestinal (GI) tract where it regulates intestinal movements, and is synthesized in serotonergic neurons of the central nervous system (CNS). It is involved in the regulation of mood, appetite, and sleep. It also has some cognitive functions, including memory and learning. Low dose serotonin is indicated in all mood disorders, depression, migraines, addictions and diet disorders. (See also **Nutrition and dieting.**)

Somatostatin 6X: Somatostatin is an inhibitory hormone that regulates the endocrine system and affects neurotransmission and cell proliferation and inhibition of the release of numerous hormones. Low dose somatostatin is indicated in: oncological diseases, cancer treatment, hyperthyroidism.

Triiodothyronine (T3) 6X: T3 is a thyroid hormone produced by the follicular cells of the thyroid gland which affects almost every physiological process in the body, including growth and development, body temperature, metabolism, and heart rate. T3 is activated by the thyroid-stimulating hormone (TSH), which is released from the pituitary gland. T3 increases the basal metabolic rate and therefore increases the body's oxygen and energy consumption. Because T4 is converted into T3 in target tissues, T3 is 3 to 5 times more active than T4.

Main indications for the use of this low dose hormone are: hypothyroidism with T3 deficiency and overweight tendency.

Thyroxine (T4) 6X: The thyroid hormone T4, just like T3, is produced by the thyroid gland and is regulated by TSH (**Thyroid-stimulating hormone)** released by the anterior pituitary gland.

T4 is converted into T3 in target tissues, therefore thyroxine is believed to be a prohormone and a reservoir for the most active and main thyroid hormone T3.

Main indications for the use of this low dose hormone are: hypothyroidism with T4 deficiency, growth disorders, physical and neurasthenia, and overweight tendency. As T4 is converted into T3, this hormone should be the first choice in thyroid target therapies.

Thyroid-stimulating hormone – TSH 6X: TSH is produced by the anterior pituitary gland. It stimulates the thyroid gland to secrete the hormone thyroxine (T4) which is then converted into the active hormone triiodothyronine (T3), which stimulates and affects many physiological processes in the body including metabolism. About 80% of this conversion is in the liver and other organs, and 20% in the thyroid itself. Main indications for the use of this low dose hormone are: thyroid stimulation, overweight tendency, obesity, short-term treatment for depression, neurasthenia, water retention and metabolic slowdown.

Main indications of low dose homeopathic cytokines (interleukins and growth factors):

Interleukin 1 – 4C: Used rarely in biotherapy, as an immune response starter and to induce a fever reaction.

Anti-Interleukin 1 – 4C: Regulates excessive production of pro-inflammatory Interleukin 1 and 6. It is indicated in acute inflammatory conditions and fever, associated with the classic anti-inflammatory remedies. It is used to slow down articular cartilage degeneration. Also useful in some autoimmune diseases as rheumatoid arthritis, thyroiditis and multiple sclerosis.

Interleukin 2 – 4C: Stimulation of T and B lymphocytes and NK cells. Regulation and stimulation of cell-mediated immune responses. A very useful cytokine in immunodeficiency conditions such as AIDS, aging, recurrent viral infections, tumors and chemotherapy.

Interleukin 3 – 4C: IL-3 stimulates the hematopoietic stem cells into myeloid progenitor cells. Indicated in hematopoietic disorders, neutropenia during and post chemotherapy, treatment of side effects of chemotherapy, radiotherapy and antiviral therapies, aplastic anemia.

Interleukin 4 – 4C: Proliferation of B lymphocytes and mast cells. Synthesis of IgG and IgE antibodies. Anti-inflammatory effect. Useful in most autoimmune diseases like diabetes type 1, rheumatoid arthritis and multiple sclerosis. It also has a pollutants' detoxifying effect.

Interleukin 7 – 4C: Proliferation of T lymphocytes especially cytotoxic T lymphocytes. It stimulates the hematopoietic stem cells into lymphoid progenitor cells. Useful in immunodeficiency conditions such as AIDS, recurrent viral infections, tumors and during chemotherapy. Also used in wound repair.

Interleukin 10 – 4C: Suppressant of most other cytokines. Regulation of the reactivity of the organism. For regulating and modulating the immunotolerance processes and the inflammatory response. Useful in most autoimmune diseases and all chronic inflammatory conditions.

Interleukin 11 – 4C: It is a pro-inflammatory cytokine. Increases platelet formation and is involved in bone formation. It is indicated in bone healing with PTH (see low dose hormones), basic regulation during immunotherapy.

Interleukin 12 – 4C: Stimulation of the NK cells and T

lymphocytes. Stimulates cell mediated immunity. Prevention of allergic manifestations, hypersensitivity and dermatitis. Useful in all immunodeficiency conditions such as AIDS and recurrent viral and bacterial infections. The most important cytokine with Interferon Gamma in cancer therapy.

Interferon Alpha – 4C: Produced by infected cells. Activation of NK cells and T lymphocytes. Antiviral activity. Cancer therapy.

Interferon Gamma – 4C: Activation of macrophages and NK cells. Reinforces T lymphocyte activity. Antiviral and highly antibacterial activity especially during the onset of infections. Master cytokine in cancer therapy and preventive for cold and flu. Antiproliferative effects.

TGF-β 1 Transforming Growth Factor Beta 1 – 4C: Suppression of the function of the T and B lymphocytes and NK cells. Involved in different stages of healing and connective tissue regeneration. Tendon, ligament and muscle repair.

GCSF Granulocyte Colony Stimulating Factor – 4C: Stimulates granulocytes (white blood cells). Triggers the reactivity and raises the sensitivity of the immune system. Useful in the initial phase of all treatments and for chronic and autoimmune diseases. Very useful in neutropenia during and post chemotherapy.

IGF 1 Insulin-like Growth Factor 1 – 4C: For the growth and maintenance of nerve tissue. Anti Age therapy. Involved in cartilage repair. Useful in metabolic syndrome and insulin resistance, obesity and high cholesterol levels.

EGF – Epidermal Growth Factor – 4C: Stimulates epithelial cells, endothelial cells and fibroblasts. Indicated in aesthetic applications to rejuvenate skin, repair sun damage, wound repair especially lacerations and burns. Gastric acidity. Stimulates angiogenesis (contraindicated in cancer).

FGF – Fibroblast Growth Factor – 4C: Stimulates new growth of blood vessels, fibroblasts and endothelial cells. Stimulates angiogenesis (contraindicated in cancer). Indicated in anti age therapy, metabolic syndrome and insulin resistance. Anti-inflammatory effect on muscle and bones.

BDNF Brain Derived Neurotrophic Factor – 4C: Neurotrophin with an effect on neurons' growth and survival. Useful in neurological damage, stress, depression, neurodegenerative diseases, Huntington's disease, Alzheimer's, Parkinson's, dementia, learning, memory and mood disorders. It is not indicated in case of migraines.

NGF Nerve Growth Factor – 4C: Neurotrophin with an effect on growth, maintenance, and survival of certain target neurons of the nervous system. Useful in neuralgic pain and neurological damage, memory, mood disorders and multiple sclerosis.

Neurotrophin 3 (NT3) – 4C: NT3 is a neurotrophic factor of the NGF (Nerve Growth Factor) family of neurotrophins. It helps to support the survival and differentiation of existing neurons, and encourages the growth and differentiation of new neurons and synapses. Action similar to BDNF.

Neurotrophin 4 (NT4) – 4C: NT4 is a neurotrophic factor in the NGF (Nerve Growth Factor) family of neurotrophins. Action similar to NT3 and BDNF.

Ciliary Neurotrophic Factor (CNTF) – 4C: CNTF is neurotrophin with an effect on the neurons where it promotes neurotransmitter synthesis. This protein is a potent survival factor for neurons and oligodendrocytes, and may be relevant in reducing tissue destruction during inflammatory attacks. Indicated in eyesight disorders, retinal degeneration, brain aging, appetite control.

Appendix II

Single homeopathic remedies included in the complex
formulas.
Their main indications according to William Boericke (1849 - 1929)
can be found at these website addresses:
http://www.homeopathiclaboratories.com/matmed/zmatmed
.php
http://www.homeopathy-help.net/Remedies/BASIC_
REMEDIES/basic.html

ABIES NIGRA
ACETYL L-CARNITINE
ACONITUM NAPELLUS
ADRENALINUM
AESCULUS HIPPOCASTANUM
ALFALFA
a-LIPOICUM ACIDUM
ALOE SOCOTRINA
ALPHA TOCOPHEROL
ALTHAEA OFFICINALIS
ALUMINA
AMBRA GRISEA
ANACARDIUM ORIENTALE
ANAS BARBARIAE
ANGELICA ARCHANGELICA
ANISUM
ANTI-INTERLEUKIN 1 ALPHA
ANTI-INTERLEUKIN 1 BETA
ANTIMONIUM CRUDUM
APIS MELLIFICA
ARALIA RACEMOSA
ARANEA DIADEMA

ARGENTUM NITRICUM
ARNICA MONTANA
ARSENICUM ALBUM
ARTERY SUIS
ASCLEPIAS VINCETOXICUM
ASCORBIC ACID
ASPERGILLUS NIGER
BELLADONNA
BELLIS PERENNIS
BERBERIS VULGARIS
BETA CAROTENE
BETA ENDORPHIN
BETA ESTRADIOL
BISMUTHUM
BONE SUIS
BRAIN DERIVED NEUROTROPHIC FACTOR -BDNF
BRYONIA ALBA
CAFFEINUM
CALCAREA CARBONICA
CALCAREA FLUORICA
CALCAREA PHOSPHORICA
CALCAREA SULPHURICA
CALCITONIN
CALENDULA OFFICINALIS
CANDIDA ALBICANS
CAPILLARY TISSUE SUIS
CARBO VEGETABILIS
CARDUUS MARIANUS
CARTILAGO SUIS
CEREBELLUM SUIS
CHAMOMILLA
CHELIDONIUM MAJUS
CHININUM
CHOLECALCIFEROL

CIMICIFUGA RACEMOSA
CIS-ACONITIC ACID
CITRICUM ACIDUM
COCCUS CACTI
COENZYME A
COENZYME Q10
COLCHICUM AUTUMNALE
COLIBACILLINUM
NATRUM MURIATICUM
COLLAGEN SUIS
COLOCYNTHIS
CONIUM MACULATUM
COPPER GLUCONATE
CORN POPPY (PAPAVER RHOEAS)
CORPUS LUTEUM SUIS
CORTEX CEREBRALIS SUIS
CROTALUS HORRIDUS
CUPRUM
DAMIANA
DEHYDROEPIANDROSTERONE
DL MALIC ACID
DOPAMINE
DROSERA
DULCAMARA
DUODENUM SUIS
ECHINACEA ANGUSTIFOLIA
ECHINACEA PURPUREA
EMBRYO SUIS
EPIDERMAL GROWTH FACTOR -EGF
EUPHORBIUM OFFICINARUM
FIBROBLAST GROWTH FACTOR -FGF
FOLIC ACID
FORMICA RUFA
FORMICUM ACIDUM

FUMARICUM ACIDUM
FUNICULUS UMBILICALIS SUIS
GALLBLADDER SUIS
GALIUM APARINE
GALPHIMIA GLAUCA
GENTIANA LUTEA
GINSENG
GLANDULA SUPRARENALIS SUIS
GLUTATHIONE
GRANULOCYTE COLONY STIMULATING FACTOR
HAMAMELIS VIRGINIANA
HEPAR SUIS
HEPAR SULFURIS
HISTAMINUM HYDROCHLORICUM
HUMULUS LUPULUS
HYDRASTIS CANADENSIS
HYPERICUM PERFORATUM
HYPOPHYSIS SUIS
HYPOTHALAMUS SUIS
IGNATIA AMARA
INFLUENZINUM
INOSITOL
INTERFERON ALPHA
INTERFERON GAMMA
INTERLEUKIN 2
INTERLEUKIN 3
INTERLEUKIN 4
INTERLEUKIN 7
INTERLEUKIN 10
INTERLEUKIN 12
IRIS VERSICOLOR
KALI CARBONICUM
KALI PHOSPHORICUM
KALMIA LATIFOLIA

KIDNEY SUIS
L-ISOLEUCINE
L-LEUCINE
L-CYSTEINE
L-LYSINE
L-METHIONINE
L-PHENYLALANINE
LACHESIS MUTUS
LEDUM PALUSTRE
LEUCINE
LEVOTHYROXIN
LILIUM TIGRINUM
LING CHIN MUSHROOM
LIPASE ENZYME
LITHIUM
LUFFA OPERCULATA
LYCOPODIUM CLAVATUM
LYMPHATIC GLAND SUIS
LYMPHATIC VESSEL SUIS
MAGNESIUM
MALIC ACID
MANGANESE
MEDULLA OSSIS SUIS
MELATONIN
MELILOTUS OFFICINALIS
MELISSA OFFICINALIS
MERCURIUS CORROSIVUS
MERCURIUS SOLUBILIS
MERCURIUS CYANATUS
METHIONINE
METHYLGLYOXAL
MILLEFOLIUM
MUCOSA NASALIS SUIS
N-ACETYLCYSTEINE

NATRUM CARBONICUM
NATRUM MURIATICUM
NATRUM OXALACETICUM
NATRUM PYRUVICUM
NATRUM SULPHURICUM
NERVE GROWTH FACTOR -NGF
NEUROTROPHIN 3
NEUROTROPHIN 4
NIACIN
NICOTINAMIDUM
NICOTINUM
NITRICUM ACIDUM
NUX VOMICA
PAEONIA OFFICINALIS
PANCREAS SUIS
PANTOTHENIC ACID
PAPAVER RHOEAS
PARATHYROID GLAND SUIS
PARIS QUADRIFOLIA
PASSIFLORA INCARNATA
PENICILLIUM NOTATUM
PETROLEUM
PHOSPHORICUM ACIDUM
PHOSPHORUS
PHYTOLACCA DECANDRA
PINEAL GLAND SUIS
PLANTAGO MAJOR
PROGESTERONE
PROLACTIN
PROPOLIS
PROTEUS
PULSATILLA
PYROGENIUM
RECTUM SUIS

REISHI MUSHROOM (Ganoderma lucidum)
RETINOL
RHEUM
RHODODENDRON CHRYSANTHUM
RHUS TOXICODENDRON
RIBOFLAVINUM
RNA
ROSA CANINA
RUSSIAN GINSENG
RUTA GRAVEOLENS
SABADILLA
SACCHARUM OFFICINALE
SALICYLICUM ACIDUM
SAMBUCUS NIGRA
SANGUINARIA CANADENSIS
SARSAPARILLA
SCROPHULARIA NODOSA
SELENIUM
SELENOMETHIONINE
SEPIA
SILICEA
SINUSITISINUM
SODIUM BICARBONATE
SODIUM CHLORIDE
SOLIDAGO VIRGAUREA
SPLEEN SUIS
SPONGIA TOSTA
STICTA PULMONARIA
STOMACH SUIS
STRONTIUM CARBONICUM
SUCCINICUM ACIDUM
SULFUR
SYMPATHETIC NERVE SUIS
SYMPHYTUM OFFICINALE

TABACUM
TARAXACUM OFFICINALE
TARTARIC ACID
THALAMUS SUIS
THIAMINUM HYDROCHLORICUM
5-HYDROXYTRYPTOPHAN
THUJA OCCIDENTALIS
THYME
THYMUS GLAND SUIS
THYROIDINUM
TOCOPHEROL
TRANSFORMING GROWTH FACTOR BETA 1 -TGF
TRYPSIN
TRYPTOPHAN
TURMERIC
TURKEY TAIL MUSHROOM (Coriolus versicolor)
TYROSINE
URETER SUIS
URINARY BLADDER SUIS
URTICA URENS
UTERUS SUIS
VACCINIUM MYRTILLUS
VALERIANA OFFICINALIS
VALINE
VEIN SUIS
VERATRUM ALBUM
VIBURNUM OPULUS
VISCUM ALBUM
VITAMIN A
VITAMIN C
VITAMIN D
VITAMIN E
ZINCUM GLUCONICUM

About the Author

Max Corradi (MBRCP, MICNM, MISOHH, Hons) was born in Milan, Italy.

Since 1996 he has been studying and practicing eastern and western philosophy, metaphysics, complementary and alternative medicine.

Interested for many years in Tibetan medicine and homeopathy, he has graduated with Honours in homeopathy and homotoxicology (complex homeopathy) at the Biomedic Centre in London. He has also received a Certificate in applied Homotoxicology from the International Academy of Homotoxicology, Baden-Baden, Germany, and has also obtained a Specialist Diploma in Physiological Regulating Medicine (PRM) at the International Academy of Physiological Regulating Medicine.

He lives and works in London, England as a Complementary and Natural Medicine Practitioner. He is a member of the British Register of Complementary Practitioners (BRCP), the Institute for Complementary and Natural Medicine (ICNM), and The International Society of Homotoxicology and Homeopathy (ISOHH).

AYNI
BOOKS

"Ayni" is a Quechua word meaning "reciprocity" – sharing, giving and receiving - whatever you give out comes back to you. To be in Ayni is to be in balance, harmony and right relationship with oneself and nature, of which we are all an intrinsic part. Complementary and Alternative approaches to health and well-being essentially follow a holistic model, within which one is given support and encouragement to move towards a state of balance, true health and wholeness, ultimately leading to the awareness of one's unique place in the Universal jigsaw of life – Ayni, in fact.